The NHS Experience

'Your son has cystic fibrosis.' The doctor said the words again, clearly expecting some kind of response. Susan stared at him, all too clear what it meant now. All she could say was 'He can't have it. Not that. . . .' The doctor interrupted, avoiding her eyes and looking down at Daniel's notes. 'I'm very sorry, Mrs Johnson, but I'm afraid he does.'

The NHS Experience is an accessible and engaging guide for all those journeying through the NHS, whether as patients, carers or professionals. It draws on the experience of staff and families at Great Ormond Street Hospital to provide good practice guidance for both users and providers of health care.

This unique book is based on the successful Snakes and Ladders drama programme developed at Great Ormond Street Hospital. It uses the story of Daniel, a fictional child with the life-limiting disease cystic fibrosis, to provide insight into the enormous challenges faced by patients, their families and the professionals involved in their care.

Asking difficult questions about how we can improve *The NHS Experience* for everyone at the front line, Daniel's story builds on information from a wealth of sources to highlight:

- The practical, ethical, resource and financial dilemmas integral to the NHS.
- The vital issues around communication, trust, management of clinical errors, consent, shared decision-making and bereavement.
- The realities of fragmented care, bed shortages, uncertain diagnoses, and complex and difficult treatment choices.

This is a book that should be read by all healthcare professionals and everyone who needs to use the NHS.

Hilary Cass is a consultant paediatrician, specialising in the care of children with disabilities. She is Deputy Medical Director at Great Ormond Street Hospital, where she is in charge of medical and multi-professional education, and is also Professor of Children's Healthcare Development at London South Bank University.

With practical insight into the patient, legal and ethical issues from **Bea Teuten**, family advocate at Great Ormond Street Hospital, and solicitor.

The NHS Experience

The 'Snakes and Ladders' guide for
patients and professionals

Hilary Cass

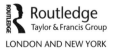
Routledge
Taylor & Francis Group

LONDON AND NEW YORK

First published 2006
by Routledge
2 Park Square, Milton Park, Abingdon, Oxon OX14 4RN

Simultaneously published in the USA and Canada
by Routledge
270 Madison Ave, New York, NY 10016

Routledge is an imprint of the Taylor & Francis Group

© 2006 Hilary Cass

Typeset in Charter and Futura by
Keystroke, Jacaranda Lodge, Wolverhampton
Printed and bound in Great Britain by
TJ International Ltd, Padstow, Cornwall

British Library Cataloguing in Publication Data
A catalogue record for this book is available from the British Library

Library of Congress Cataloging in Publication Data
A catalog record for this book has been requested

ISBN10: 0–415–33671–6   ISBN13: 9–78–0–415–33671–0 (pbk)

Any resemblance between the fictional characters mentioned or
portrayed in the extracts relating to Daniel and his family and any
living or actual persons is purely coincidental. Information obtained
from this text is intended to supplement, but not substitute for
professional care. If you have or suspect you have a problem, you
should seek appropriate clinical advice.

Contents

Illustrations

Figures

Tables

Boxes

Abbreviations

A&E	Accident and Emergency
ANH	artifical nutrition and hydration
BMA	British Medical Association
BMJ	*British Medical Journal*
CCN	community children's nurse
CNST	Clinical Negligence Scheme for Trusts
CSP	clinical site practitioner
DNA	did not attend
DNAR	Do not attempt resuscitation
EWTD	European Working Time Directive
GMC	General Medical Council
GOSH	Great Ormond Street Hospital
GP	general practitioner
ICAS	Independent Complaints Advocacy Service
IVF	in-vitro fertilisation
NHS	National Health Service
NICE	National Institute of Clinical Excellence
NPSA	National Patient Safety Agency
NRLS	National Reporting and Learning System
NSF	National Service Frameworks
OECD	Organisation for Economic Cooperation and Development
PALS	Patient Advice and Liaison Service
PCG	Primary Care Group
PCT	Primary Care Trust
PDP	personal development plan
PiP	Partners in Paediatrics
PVS	permanent vegetative state
QALY	quality adjusted life year
RCT	randomised controlled trial
SHA	Strategic Health Authority

Foreword

All health professionals need a combination of skills that includes the ability to communicate, observe, diagnose, treat and care for their patients. The balance of skills varies between the different professions, but all need to be able to communicate with patients and, in the case of children, their families too. Disappointingly, it is this skill, or rather lack of it, which is often found wanting when patients or their families complain. Recognising this need led to the development of a monthly programme of interactive sessions for health professionals from all disciplines called 'Snakes and Ladders' at Great Ormond Street Hospital NHS Trust. A combination of staff and actors played the parts, and challenging scenarios were played out. What it achieved particularly well was a sense of what it feels like to be the parent or child receiving information. Communication, which is a two-way process, couldn't start until the initial shock had worn off and trust on both sides had developed. It became clear during some of the episodes that health professionals were informing, not communicating with, the family and yet were totally unaware of this mismatch between what they thought they were doing and what the family really needed and wanted. The Snakes and Ladders project helped bring this lesson home, but it also showed how difficult it is to achieve, because of the way health care is now delivered. There is much greater potential for the child and family to experience health care as a series of disjointed episodes, where there is no time for relationships to develop. For individuals with chronic health problems, this is clearly a major problem.

There are many ways to overcome this fragmentation: for example, the role of nurse specialists is particularly important. This book gives a bigger audience the chance to consider the issues. They weren't always comfortable for us at GOSH, as they held up a mirror to some of our practices in a less than favourable way. You may find the book uncomfortable too if you are a health professional. We hope all readers will find the book useful – after all, we all use health services at some time.

Jane Collins
Chief Executive, Great Ormond Street Hospital

Preface

The Snakes and Ladders project

It was 1 October 1998. The sign on the door of the office said 'Director of Postgraduate Medical Education'. I stepped inside and, after some hesitation, sat down at the desk. The bookshelves were empty, the walls were bare and a rapid inventory of the desk drawer revealed a stapler, a hole punch, three discarded paper clips and the tail end of a packet of Polos. I carefully reread the handover notes from my predecessor and wondered what to do next. Investigating the in-tray, I found two study-leave applications that needed my signature and a letter from the Postgraduate Dean, congratulating me on my new appointment. As I read her letter, I felt a growing sense of panic at the task I had undertaken. Suddenly I had overall responsibility for the education and welfare of every junior doctor who passed through the doors of Great Ormond Street Hospital (GOSH) – the largest children's hospital in the country, with a national and international reputation as a major teaching centre.

I need not have worried. On a day-to-day basis, my 'charges' were taught their craft by some of the foremost specialists in the country. I merely had to conduct an extremely well-rehearsed orchestra. But, as time went on, I started to worry about the broader, more holistic aspects of their education. The NHS was changing. So were patient expectations – and rightly so. It was no longer enough for doctors to have excellent technical skills in diagnosis or treatment. As explained by Jane Collins in the foreword to this book, unless they could also develop the ability to communicate effectively, to function collaboratively in teams and to understand the political and societal pressures within which they worked, they would face stress, litigation and failure. Worse still, they would not be effective in meeting the needs of the patients and families they were committed to treating.

Criticising doctors for their failure to communicate has become something of a national preoccupation, but the problems are more complex and profound, and they affect not only doctors, but all staff working within the NHS. Nurses, therapists, pharmacists, managers: all need to work within a stretched and politicised system, but at the same time maintain an understanding of the patient's perspective. Fly-on-the-wall documentaries and reality television demonstrate that people identify best with problems when they are personalised. This presents a dilemma. Health-care staff have to learn not to over-identify with their patients if they are to maintain a professional approach, but at the same time they need to be able to put themselves in their shoes in order to understand and improve on system failures. With this in mind, I hit on the idea of using professional role players to dramatise the story of a fictional child from infancy through to adolescence, using his journey through the health-care system to illustrate the problems and pitfalls and to facilitate discussion about possible solutions.

With Francina Cunnington, the Senior Education Lead in my department, I set up a multi-professional project team involving doctors, nurses, managers, therapists, our Head Pharmacist, Press Office, Medical Illustration Department and a professional role-play company – and we embarked on the task of devising our storyline. Getting agreement between two parents when naming a child is difficult enough; our hero had fifteen vocal and committed parents! But, despite the early labour pains, the team successfully gave birth to Daniel, our fictional patient, and the first episode of 'Snakes and Ladders: Learning About the Ups and Downs of the Patient Journey' went live on 11 September 2002.

Two further people were crucial to the success of the Snakes and Ladders project – both on stage, and in the writing of this book. The first was Bea Teuten, a family-law solicitor with a Master's in medical ethics and law from King's College, London. Bea has a daughter who was born with congenital toxoplasmosis, a condition that can result in neurological, visual and hearing problems. In 1989 she founded a medical charity 'The Toxoplasmosis Trust' and was Chair until 2000. She thus has first-hand experience of the problems facing children and their carers in navigating the Health Service; at one stage, her daughter, a GOSH patient, was under the care of seven consultants at one time! In 2002, Bea came back to Great Ormond Street in a new guise and set up the PALS (Patient Advice and Liaison Service), working with children, their families and clinical teams to help resolve a vast array of issues, including treatment and end-of-life decisions. Bea rapidly became a key member of the Snakes and Ladders team, offering a first-hand patient perspective as the drama evolved and alerting us to 'hot issues' for parents who were presenting through the PALS office.

The second key player was Dr Sophie Petit-Zeman, who was then working in the Press Office at GOSH. Sophie has a background in neuroscience research and mental health, communications and journalism, and is a council member of the Brain and Spine Foundation. She has also worked in the NHS, private and voluntary sectors, in the UK and abroad. As well as bringing a personal perspective to the development of the storyline as a member of the project team, Sophie's extensive experience as a journalist and science writer made Daniel Johnson something of a celebrity, both within the hospital and externally. The Snakes and Ladders story featured in *Roundabout* (the GOSH magazine), on the GOSH intranet and on our external web site. Audiences grew to include clinicians from other hospitals, general practitioners (GPs) and a range of other visitors, including the Deputy Chief Medical Officer. Sophie went on to produce a series of articles in the nursing, medical and public press and was instrumental in Snakes and Ladders being awarded a runner-up prize in the Health Service Journal Awards. When Sophie suggested that Snakes and Ladders should be translated from stage to page, I was highly dubious, but was won over by her conviction that the project was possible. This book has therefore drawn on a unique combination of skills and knowledge: my perspective as a doctor and educator, Bea's input to the 'learning points for patients', and to the legal and ethical discussions, and early help and advice from Sophie, as a medical journalist.

The Snakes and Ladders project is ongoing. The stage version has now been translated onto DVD, and Francina Cunnington is now leading on translating the material into an accredited teaching programme that we hope will be more widely available in the near future.

Hilary Cass
March 2005

Acknowledgements

Many people have contributed, in varied and invaluable ways, to the creation of this book. The author would like to thank the whole Snakes and Ladders team: Paul Aurora, Sarah Bonham, Julia Chisholm, Jude Cope, Finella Craig, Francina Cunnington, Robert Dinwiddie, Phill Doulton, Maureen Ferguson, Nick Geddes, Ann Goldman, Quen Mok, Jean Simons, Isabel Smith, Bea Teuten, Vivian Whitaker and Pauline Whitmore.

As explained in the Preface, particular thanks are due to Bea Teuten and Sophie Petit-Zeman. Bea's unique insight as a patient advocate, parent, lawyer and medical ethicist and Sophie's perspective as a science writer and journalist have enriched 'Snakes and Ladders' enormously – both on stage and in print.

I am also very grateful to Francina Cunnington, whose commitment to the Snakes and Ladders project helped turn it from a pipe dream into a reality. She is now developing the material into a teaching programme, which will soon be available through a number of higher-education institutions.

Another important perspective has been brought by Tracey and Keith McBride. Their willingness to revisit some of the more painful aspects of caring for a child with complex health needs and to share their insight into the health-care system has been both humbling and generous and is a tribute to the memory of their daughter Katie.

When enmeshed in a project such as this one, it is easy to lose perspective and consistency of approach. I would like to thank Sally Carr for working tirelessly through this manuscript and for ensuring that the style remained readable and accessible throughout.

I would like to thank two of my nursing colleagues: Judith Ellis, who spent several summer afternoons in my back garden, deliberating on how to distil a challenge as huge and complex as the NHS into a few short chapters, and Michelle Johnson who ensured that Penny was a credible and creditable reflection of community children's nurse practice.

Finally, I would like to thank Jane Collins, Chief Executive at Great Ormond Street Hospital, for supporting this project in its journey from stage to page.

Acknowledgements are due to the Healthcare Commission for Figure 3.1, to the Modernisation Agency for Table 4.1 and to the *British Medical Journal* for Table 6.1.

This book is dedicated to all the children, families and staff at Great Ormond Street Hospital – past, present and future.

1 Beginnings

Wednesday lunchtime at the Albion Children's Hospital. A heavy autumnal sky dulls the out-patient area, where Susan Johnson, her husband Matthew and their six-week-old son Daniel are waiting to see the doctor. An abandoned newspaper on the chair beside Susan carries the headline 'NHS Rocked by Organ Scandal'. She doesn't want to read it, but needs something to take her mind off the wait. She chats briefly to the mother of a very noisy toddler who has already had two tantrums in the past half hour and looks set to launch into a third. Somehow this makes things worse. Susan can't help thinking that the other little boy looks so well, and she's sure that there's something seriously wrong with Daniel. Once again, she pulls out his baby book and tries to convince herself that his painfully slow weight gain is just down to his stormy first weeks in hospital. That it will soon pick up.

In a small room across the corridor, Dr Sebastian Hill is feeling nervous. He knows there's a family waiting to see him – the Johnsons – but he stalls for time by refiling an X-ray report that is out of sequence. All in all, it's beginning to feel like 'one of those days'. He was even late starting this clinic because he was delayed on the ward helping a junior colleague put a drip up on a child with severe asthma. Then things got progressively more behind while he waited for an interpreter for his first patient and spent some time chasing up an important test result on the next patient. Now he's about to tell the Johnsons that their son has a serious life-shortening illness, and the specialist nurse who would normally have been there to break the news with him has called in sick. Sebastian is just one week into his first teaching-hospital registrar job, and he knows he should probably ask his consultant for help. But after calling her twice already this morning, he desperately wants to make a good impression by getting through the rest of the clinic independently.

The sound of a drill starts up again outside, from the site of the new hospital wing. Daniel starts to cry. Matthew tells Susan it's outrageous that the wait's so long. Sebastian closes the window to try to block out at least some of the drilling noise before calling the Johnsons in, though it's unbearably muggy since the heating goes automatically to high in September. Glancing across at the new building, blue tarpaulin flapping from its scaffolding, Sebastian wonders fleetingly whether sinking eight million pounds into a gene-therapy centre is really the best use of resources. Surely what the hospital really needs is more nurses, a better cleaning service, more interpreters to translate for those who don't speak English and a new computer system in Outpatients. Gene therapy doesn't seem very utilitarian, set against all that. But that's not his problem right now. His more immediate concern is the anxious family on the other side of the consulting-room door. So he washes his hands, glancing in the mirror as he does so, straightens his tie and gathers up Daniel's notes. Then he walks into the reception area to find the Johnsons.

It's about people

The NHS (National Health Service) occupies a curious position in the hearts and minds of the British public. It is, at the same time, both one of its proudest institutions and a 'political football'; an institution in which everyone has a stake, and about which everyone has an opinion. Health care is everybody's business.

The recent high-profile cases and increasing politicisation of the Health Service have made its public face too often one of errors, waiting-list crises, 'organ scandals' and managerial obfuscation. Yet, despite the media interest and spin associated with these events, public confidence in doctors remains higher than in any other professional group. Most service users remain positive about their experiences of health care, and NHS staff report high personal satisfaction with their jobs.

How can these apparently differing perspectives be reconciled? The answer lies with the people who sit at the heart of this book: the people who use the NHS and who rightly expect to be seen by health-care staff who communicate effectively, perform their roles competently and treat them with respect; and the people who staff the NHS and face the challenge of providing that health care within the financial and organisational constraints of a large and complex system.

While government policy, funding arrangements, policy statements and star ratings are impersonal, the people at the end of the waiting lists are real. What matters – and what ultimately leaves a lasting impression on both parties – is the interaction that takes place between the patient and the doctor, nurse, physiotherapist or pharmacist responsible for their care. The vast NHS machinery that brought them into a room together suddenly fades from view, and the success or failure of the interaction then moves into the hands of those individuals.

The impetus to write this book arose from a dramatic and unique approach to personalising these issues in order to improve patient care at Great Ormond Street Hospital for Children (GOSH). Called 'Snakes and Ladders: Learning about the Ups and Downs of the Patient Journey', it was a new departure in medical and multi-professional education. Across the country and, indeed, the world, doctors are familiar with the hospital 'Grand Round': a rite of passage in which juniors present a clever diagnosis, a cutting-edge piece of research, the latest information about their subject to an audience of peers and seniors. One lunchtime in September 2002 (while doubtless countless families waited just like the Johnsons and doctors like Sebastian tried to prepare themselves for a difficult consultation), the Grand Round was reborn. Professional role players were brought into the hospital lecture theatre to play out the story of one fictional young patient from birth, through his illness, to wherever his adolescence and the tale led. Staff participated in, and were encouraged to influence and criticise, this hour-long monthly drama, which was aimed at all 'front-line' clinicians, managers, secretaries and a variety of other support staff – everyone working at GOSH – because improving the experience of patients and families depends on them all. The audience was given the opportunity to work through the practical, clinical, ethical and emotional challenges confronting the Johnsons, Sebastian Hill and the other staff involved in Daniel's care. And, despite the fact that staff had their fill of the day-to-day drama of hospital life in every moment of their working day and could top up, if desired, with an extra fix of *Casualty* or *ER* in the evening, they came in droves to spend one lunchtime a month keeping up with the Johnsons. It was a far more effective way of communicating important issues than reading the latest policies on drug safety, consent or bed management.

But it is not enough to have just played out the issues with the staff who came into the lecture theatre and with visiting colleagues from district general hospitals and primary care. We also need to extend the messages to staff working across the NHS, whether in paediatric settings, in adult care, in acute trusts or in the community – because the core principles of patient-centred care are important to us all. And if the messages are about patient-centred care, it is crucial that we also share them with the many Daniels, now in their teens or young adulthood, and with their parents, grandparents, siblings and friends. With the many people at all ages and stages who use the NHS on a day-to-day basis and who wish to understand what makes it tick, how to get the best out of it and how to help improve it. This book thus replays the journey that we at GOSH, and frequent professional external visitors, followed on stage, in debate, on-line and through printed back-up material after each episode.

It's about time

Daniel Johnson was 'born' on 1 August 2002, shortly after the NHS celebrated its fifty-fourth birthday. Through the greater part of that half century, health care in general and the medical profession in particular operated through a benevolent paternalism, largely accepted by the public because of the perceived expertise and dedication of its practitioners.

The first seeds of cultural change started to emerge through Thatcher's consumerist approach of the 1980s. The Labour Government that gave birth to the NHS had predicted that costs would fall as the service improved the health of the nation. The naivety of that prediction became all too obvious in a very short time and continued to vex successive governments. And so it was that in 1989 the Conservative Government published its White Paper *Working for Patients*, which attempted to drive quality improvement and greater economic control through the development of an 'internal market'. Health care and medical treatment became commodities: purchased by local health authorities and GPs from hospitals restyled as independent trusts, all supposedly working together in the best interests of the new 'consumer'. Unfortunately, capacity problems beset the best intentions of the reforms, and quality was soon overridden by financial constraint and cost containment. It rapidly became apparent that well-trained staff, good facilities and modern equipment do not automatically converge to create high standards of health care. Disaster struck, and serious failings in care standards hit the headlines through the early to mid-1990s. Where was the quality-assurance framework overseeing the work of trusts now in financial competition with each other?

In January 1995, a child called Joshua Loveday died at the Bristol Royal Infirmary after major heart surgery. This might have been viewed as a sad, but not very remarkable event were it not for the fact that Joshua died in a unit with a track record of unacceptably poor outcomes after such surgery. And, despite the fact that the Trust Senior Management was already aware of the outcome data and the need for significant service changes, Joshua's surgery still went ahead – with tragic results.

The crisis in paediatric cardiac surgery in Bristol was the first of a series of high-profile cases that was to set the scene for a major change in Health Service philosophy. The Government White Paper *The New NHS: Modern, Dependable* (Department of Health 1997), closely followed by its sister paper *A First Class Service* (Department of Health 1998), continued the Conservative Administration's theme of patient-centred care, but abolished the internal market in favour of a quality-driven model based on the principles of 'clinical governance'. This is the framework through which NHS organisations must improve the quality of their services and safeguard high standards.

As Chief Medical Officer Liam Donaldson wrote in the *Journal of Epidemiology and Community Health* (Donaldson 1998: 73)

> A frequently aired concern of health professionals throughout the world is the extent to which financial issues dominate the health care agenda. If most of the time of the senior management of health care organisations is directed towards finance . . . how can a commitment towards quality be anything other than rhetoric?

And, speaking at an international symposium (Donaldson 1999), he highlighted the extent to which public expectations of the NHS also lie behind the changes. 'Rising patient and public expectations are becoming a key stimulus to improving quality in the NHS. People – particularly those under 45 years – are less ready than in the past to accept a paternalistic style of service from the NHS.'

It's about change

A philosophical and cultural sea change was clearly crucial, but was far from being the only development need. The NHS Plan (NHS Executive 2000) recognised under-investment and staffing shortfalls within the Health Service and set ambitious targets to remedy these. But while the promise to employ 7,500 more consultants, 2,000 more

GPs, 20,000 more nurses and 6,500 more therapists is laudable, many questions remain unanswered: Where will extra staff come from? Who will train them? and How can resources keep pace with the extra investigations and procedures that a larger workforce would inevitably generate? Targets to cut junior doctors' hours are seen as vital in ensuring that patients are not treated by doctors who are too tired to work safely, but how can this be reconciled with training needs – spending enough hours on the job to learn how to do it? What about the knock-on effect for consultants whose hours are less rigorously controlled?

As waiting-list targets multiply and public expectations escalate, alongside promises of increased choice about treatment dates and places, do we need more health-care centres and hospitals, or will this spread limited resources too thin? How can the convenience of local care be weighed up against the benefits of centralising services in a smaller number of large specialist centres? What do patients really want? and How can we get answers to all these questions?

This book confronts real issues using a fictionalised account to illustrate generic topics. A central tenet of the book is that in almost every health-care episode there are three aspects to consider: the health-care system within which the action takes place; the societal context, be it political, cultural, financial or ethical; and the actions of the people at the front line, both patients and staff.

Each of the remaining chapters of the book is divided into two main parts. The first tells the Johnsons' story, whilst the second analyses the issues and discusses how the most visible end point – the interaction between patients and staff – is influenced by the system and societal climate, which is the crucible within which that interaction takes place (see Figure 1.1). A closing section entitled 'At the End of the Day', uses the main fictional characters to explore outstanding points of tension, to highlight areas that remain particularly difficult to resolve, or simply to set out open questions. The book does not seek to prescribe neat, unrealistic cures for intractable health-care problems, but to open up the issues and discussion points. Learning points for both staff and patients are given throughout each chapter.

For those at the front line, whether staff or patients, part of the frustration when things go wrong is that they feel impotent to change or improve things. The health-care system seems like such a large and incomprehensible machine that no one individual can influence it. In reality, understanding the system and the broader context is important for a number of reasons:

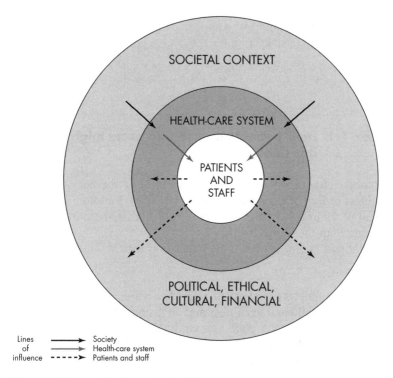

Figure 1.1 Lines of influence in health care.

- First, because it allows those at the front line, both staff and patients, to make better sense of the situations in which they find themselves.
- Second, because it allows them not only to focus on the issues that they can influence most strongly, but also to understand that failings are not always the fault of the individuals most directly involved.
- Third, and perhaps most importantly, because local systems and processes are driven both externally and internally – externally by the broader political and financial agenda and internally by the individuals taking part in those processes. It is people who can and do change local systems – and who can sometimes even have an impact on the much larger political horizon, as the Kennedy Report, *Learning from Bristol* (Bristol Royal Infirmary Inquiry 2001), so clearly demonstrates.

A small body of determined spirits fired by an unquenchable faith in their mission can alter the course of history.

(Mahatma Gandhi)

Box 1.1 How patients and service users might use this book

Illness is frequently a frightening experience, whether our own illness or that of close friends and loved ones. But often it is the fear of the unknown and the lack of control that are more frightening than the illness itself.

Patients and members of the public may use this book in three ways:

1 At its simplest level, it will provide a window onto the story of one child and his illness and an insight into the complexities of providing good and equitable health care, whether in the NHS or any other health-care system.

2 Equally importantly, it will help users to understand what they might reasonably expect of the NHS, how to take some control over the outcome of their own care and, perhaps, even to participate in changing and improving local health-care systems through patient involvement forums.

3 Finally, it will give users a better understanding of the perspective of the Health Service staff whom they encounter on their journey through the NHS.

Box 1.2 How health-care professionals might use this book

Staff within the NHS often feel just as powerless as the patients they serve – not because of the uncertainty of illness, but because of the confusing and sometimes conflicting array of directives that they are expected to follow, the increasing demands of the public and the resource pressures within which they work.

For staff, just as for patients, better understanding is also an essential prerequisite to better control.

Health-care professionals may use this book in three ways:

1 To develop a clearer understanding of the broader context of the Health Service within which they work.
2 To find better ways of managing the clinical and practical situations within which they find themselves and to influence the systems within which they work.
3 To better understand the perspective of the patients for whom they provide support and clinical care.

By focusing on the problems faced by one child and his family, the book necessarily highlights the negative in order to suggest and explore solutions. Descriptions of seamless and efficient health-care delivery do not make exciting reading, and, more importantly, do not carry the key lessons that this book hopes to convey. For families of children with cystic fibrosis – and indeed for all health-care users – it is important to understand that Daniel's journey is not typical but provides a pot-pourri of the potential pitfalls in health care, in order to help readers – regardless of which side of the 'NHS desk' they sit – to make it better.

2 It's not what you say

The diagnosis

The Johnsons

Daniel was nearly two weeks old when Susan and Matthew finally brought him home from hospital. The first time she carried him into the living room, Susan found herself focusing on trivial and irrelevant details, as if seeing them for the first time: the crack in the tile over the fireplace, Sara's Barbie-pink school bag, the plant that Matthew had forgotten to water in her absence. She'd expected to be away from home for two days, and she'd spent just one night here in the past two weeks. That was when Matthew had insisted that she entrusted Daniel to him – and of course the nurses – and spent a night in her own bed to try and catch up on some sleep.

During the first few hours of Daniel's life, Susan had told Matthew that he was very different from Sara – now ten, and memorable for having been the 'perfect baby'. 'Typical boy,' she'd said. 'Doesn't stay still for a moment.' But as he had continued to wriggle uncomfortably in her arms and to scream inconsolably, she had felt a growing sense of dread, which she tried to suppress by telling herself that she was being neurotic because he was such a precious baby.

Susan was the youngest of seven children from an Irish Catholic family. They had moved to southern England when she was four. Her first marriage to Tariq, an Asian Muslim from Manchester, ended when their daughter Sara was two years old. Susan was furious that her family saw this as a vindication of their objections to the marriage and was too proud and stubborn to ask them for financial help. So she continued to hold down a secretarial job whilst raising two-year-old Sara by herself.

She met Matthew at a school reunion soon afterwards; he was four years her junior, and she didn't remember him at all. She confessed that she'd come to the party because her social life had evaporated with the advent of single-parenthood; he admitted he didn't know why he'd come at all, as he'd always hated the place and had been bullied. Shy and self-effacing, the only child of a quiet Scottish couple who were both music teachers, Matthew was everything Tariq hadn't been. They were married six months later.

Matthew was a steadfast partner and was very good with Sara. But sometimes Susan felt she was mothering two children. She hoped that having a child of their own would equalise their relationship a bit more, so she was quite unprepared for the seven-year gap during which she couldn't conceive. Months of arguments about whether they should try IVF (in-vitro fertilisation) ended in sudden jubilation when she discovered she was pregnant with Daniel.

The Albion Children's Hospital

It had taken forty-eight hours of failing to persuade Daniel to feed whilst bizarrely his tummy seemed to be ballooning, before the doctors had dropped their bombshell. One minute Daniel had been taken off for an X-ray and the next they were arranging to have him transferred from St Michael's to the Albion Children's Hospital for surgery.

Susan had seen the Albion on the television; it was forever in the news for things like gene therapy and complicated transplants. The hospital was nowhere near where they lived and, as the doctors and nurses at St Michael's had all seemed busy getting Daniel ready for the journey, there had been no one Susan could ask about why he had to go. Or what the surgery was for.

A very young-looking doctor had said something earlier about how the X-ray showed that Daniel had 'meconium ileus,' and about needing to relieve a blockage. Susan hadn't understood, but then the doctor's bleep had gone off, and anyway she'd felt a bit daunted, afraid to bother him with questions. In desperation, she resolved to talk to one of the nurses a bit later, but later never came.

Daniel and Susan had arrived at the Albion at 8.30 p.m. that night. When Matthew arrived an hour later, after dropping Sara off with a neighbour, Susan hadn't told him about the conversation she had just overheard between the doctor and one of the nurses. About cystic fibrosis. About how hard it was to imagine being a parent of a newborn getting the diagnosis. She had no idea whether they thought Daniel had cystic fibrosis or were talking about another child on the ward.

Cystic fibrosis. She was sure that was what the girl at school had died of. She was in Susan's class, four years older than Matthew, so he wouldn't remember her. And, anyway, she had made up her mind that the doctor definitely couldn't have been talking about them, about Daniel, so there was absolutely no point in worrying Matthew.

After the operation, the staff had been very reassuring, telling her how well it had gone, and Daniel had started feeding properly. Susan stayed with him on the ward for another ten days, and then they'd done some more blood tests and had sent him home. They said his stitches would just dissolve, but that he needed to come back for a follow-up appointment. Susan supposed it was to check that he was still well. They let them go home without any special advice and, certainly, no one seemed worried.

Her sense of relief only lasted for two weeks; by the third she was scared again. Daniel wasn't growing. Matthew told Susan he had read that babies lost weight at the beginning. The health visitor came, nodded with approval as she watched Daniel feed and reassured Susan that his slow weight gain was probably because he had been so ill at first and that he would soon catch up. She had promised to have a word with the GP about Daniel and to see if he'd had a report from the Albion.

Susan wasn't reassured. She had rung the hospital one day when Matthew was at work – she didn't want him to think she was being silly – but no one knew who could help. When they asked her what was wrong with her son, why he had been there, what operation he'd had, she didn't know. She felt stupid, and totally lost.

The diagnosis

Daniel's appointment letter finally came through, and Susan and Matthew took him back to the Albion. Susan was so relieved when the day came, but once they got there the wait to be seen was more than an hour. Susan wondered if they had made a mistake with the appointment, because this seemed to be a medical rather than a surgical outpatient department. None of the other children waiting had had an operation recently.

When the doctor finally came to get them, he had a file in his hand and looked in it for Daniel's name, after trying 'Damien'. The stethoscope around his neck made him look important, but when he shook Susan's hand, the black and silver bit at the end banged Daniel's face. Susan wondered why he bothered wearing the stethoscope at all, as that was the closest he got to Daniel in the whole meeting.

Susan couldn't remember exactly when he first said 'cystic fibrosis', but as soon as he did all she could think about was that schoolfriend again. Amy, that was it. It was years ago, but suddenly Susan was back in the assembly hall, a tall room marked out for badminton, climbing ropes hanging from the walls next to the gym bars, the headmistress on a stage at the end. It was the first day of the Christmas term, and the headmistress had started with the announcements: Class 5 music exams next week so don't forget your recorders; no one excused from games without a note from their parents; any school library books taken out before the holidays must be back by Friday. And then, after a heavy pause, the headmistress telling them that Amy had died. Died of cystic fibrosis. So now, when Susan heard the words again, she was back there in the school gym, staring at the tall grimy windows, the climbing ropes, the bars, the coloured plastic cones stacked up at the side.

'. . . cystic fibrosis.' The doctor said the words again, and looked from her to Matthew and back again, clearly expecting some kind of response. Susan dragged herself back to the present and stared at him, all too clear what it meant now, all these years later. Matthew didn't react, and all she could say was 'He can't. He can't have it, not that . . .'

The doctor interrupted, avoiding her eyes and looking down at Daniel's notes. 'I'm very sorry, but I'm afraid he does.'

Matthew stared at the doctor too. At the badge that said 'Dr Sebastian Hill, SpR Respiratory', and wondered what SpR meant. And then fixed his eyes on where the stethoscope was wrinkling Dr Hill's shirt collar, on his tie with pictures of sheep on it and what looked like an egg stain. No one spoke, and a drill started up outside. The noise outside only made the silence in the room seem interminable.

Then Dr Hill started to talk very fast, words tumbling out like a fast-flowing stream: 'The meconium ileus op was just a first step, symptomatic relief, getting rid of the baby poo that was bunging him up. Then the sweat test showed plenty of salt, so it was really no surprise that the blood screens confirmed the genetic mutation. It really was a huge step, cloning and characterising the CF transmembrane conductance regulator gene, back in, oh I don't know, the early 90s I think. Just such a shame you're both carriers . . . bad luck . . . So your Dan's got the deltaF508 mutation . . . But you don't want to get bogged down in biology . . . Anyway, he's such a lovely baby . . . your first child? . . . May be ways we can help you have another who'll be normal . . . For Dan, there's every chance of a good childhood ahead, maybe more . . . can't cure it, it's in his cells, but can manage it . . . regular physiotherapy . . . enzymatic replacement, I think . . . I need to talk to colleagues a bit, not been here long myself . . .'

Susan wondered whether to point out that Daniel wasn't her first child, but she didn't dare. Not in front of Matthew. They had had a terrible row on the day of Daniel's operation, when Matthew had said that all this was easier for her because she already had Sara. As if that would have made any difference to her grief if Daniel hadn't survived the surgery. She certainly didn't want to reopen that scar, but nonetheless she did want to ask why Sara wasn't affected, until it occurred to her that Sara might get it or maybe she had it without them knowing? And what did Dr Hill mean about helping them to have another child who'd be well? Wasn't that a bit like Matthew saying how having Sara made it all easier for Susan? Couldn't any of them see how she was in so much pain about *this* little boy? And anyway, how could they arrange for any other child to be OK? How could they be so sure? And how ill was Daniel? She looked down at him, asleep in her arms and managed not to wake him as she scrabbled in her handbag for a tissue.

Dr Hill spoke across the painful silence, '. . . Infertility's always a problem. For him, the boy I mean. But that's really not to worry you now of course. And anyway, chances are he may reach an almost normal young adulthood.' And then he leant forward in his chair, glanced again at Daniel's notes and asked if there was anything they didn't understand.

Dr Sebastian Hill

Sebastian Hill's parents were surprised when he told them he wanted to become a doctor. As a child he had always had his nose in a book, had nagged them into taking him to the Science Museum on numerous occasions and, for as long as they could remember, had been fascinated by physics and astronomy. His father was an academic chemist, and everyone was convinced that Sebastian would follow him down the pure science route.

His mother, who had been a GP for several years before giving up to look after the children full time, was worried about his decision. Not because she didn't think he would make a good doctor, but because she hoped that this wasn't a naïve response to the death of her own mother following a late diagnosis of ovarian cancer. But, despite her reservations, Sebastian really did seem clear about his decision, and he got into medical school without difficulty.

For Sebastian himself, success in exams and at work had always come remarkably easily. He surfed through medical school without doing too much work, then drifted through a number of senior house officer jobs before opting for a career in paediatrics. In line with his parents' hunch, he had long since decided that he wanted to become an academic rather than a pure clinician, but for the first time in his life had hit a brick wall when he didn't manage to get funding for a Ph.D. project.

Five minutes into Sebastian's meeting with the Johnsons, he knew he was out of his depth and was handling it appallingly badly. He reflected on the fact that he was off form because he'd had a row with his girlfriend the night before, was feeling nervous about his new job and, to cap it all, had just heard that yet another grant proposal application had been rejected. But he also knew that none of this was any excuse for slipping into incomprehensible jargon, for communicating so ineptly, for even having embarked on the consultation single-handedly. And, as he headed for the canteen at the end of his clinic, the sight of the Johnsons sitting in the pharmacy waiting area, Susan sobbing silently into a sodden tissue, Matthew with his arm round her shoulder, made him wish he could start the day again.

Cut! Rewind

Sebastian wanted to replay his day. One of the most appealing aspects of acting out the Snakes and Ladders drama on stage was that it was possible to do just that. The audience could ask to have the role play rerun in any way they wanted. We can't do that in real life, and, even if we could, it is rare that changing the actions of one individual can be a panacea for the problems that occur. What ultimately went wrong in our scenario was the communication between Sebastian and the Johnsons. However, as explained in Chapter 1, in almost every situation, the interactions of individuals are just the end point of a much broader cultural, ethical or political agenda and of a complex health-care system.

In this first analysis, I will illustrate how the journey that brought three adults and a small baby together so disastrously in a small consulting room on a wet autumn afternoon began many years earlier. For Dr Hill it started the day he showed his parents his offer letter to medical school, a bright young man setting out on his chosen career path. For Susan, the memory that was to shape her response to the news of her son's illness was laid down in a distant school hall when she heard of the death of a half-remembered friend. For Matthew, the devastation of the news was rooted in his long wait for his first child. And for Daniel, a tiny genetic glitch, a fault in the blueprint for life passed on to him unwittingly by both his parents, was the legacy that was to irrevocably change all their lives. And uniting all this, the Albion. A busy hospital struggling to do the right thing by patients and staff, succeeding for much of the time, but sometimes falling short amidst the conflicting pressures and resource issues that are the legacy of today's NHS.

THE HEALTH-CARE SYSTEM: UNDERSTANDING SYSTEM COMPLEXITY

Before even embarking on an analysis of the interaction in the consulting room between Dr Hill and the Johnsons, it is very important to spend some time thinking about the broader events and issues that were to set the backdrop for the consultation itself.

Hospitals such as the Albion and St Michael's are under unprecedented pressure. The Albion is GOSH's fictional alter ego. It offers the same care, faces the same challenges and its corridors throng with the same staff and patient mix. An intricately woven series of processes carry ill children through clinics and wards towards cure or treatment. Awe-inspiring gene therapy and life-saving transplants go on in a framework that must also ensure that outpatient appointments happen on time, floors are cleaned, broken light bulbs changed.

The challenge of complex systems

The London Hospital for Sick Children

WANTED for the above Institution a Matron, She must be a Member of the Church of England, single and without encumbrances and between the ages of 30/45. Salary £40 p.a. with board and lodging.

(Advert dated 21 November 1851,
in Twistington Higgins 1952: 23)

From simplicity to complexity

On 17 February 1852, 49 Great Ormond Street opened its doors to its first patient, Eliza Armstrong, a three-and-a-half-year-old with 'consumption'. The hospital boasted ten beds, two medical officers, one surgeon, a matron (whose appointment did not quite meet today's Equal Opportunities standards!), an unsalaried resident doctor, a dispenser and a secretary. In its first year, 143 inpatients were admitted and 1,250 children were seen in Outpatients. The management structure was simple: a small medical committee met weekly and kept close tabs on expenditure. For example, the purchase of a 20-gallon cask of cod-liver oil was sanctioned, 'if it would appear, as was believed, that a saving of one-third of the price would be thereby effected' (Twistington Higgins 1952: 25).

GOSH now employs almost 3,000 staff, manages an annual budget of 190 million pounds and works alongside a cutting-edge research institute. Nearly 12,000 inpatients, 7,000 day-case patients and 80,000 outpatients with rare and complicated conditions converge on GOSH annually from across the country and the world. Committees, clinicians and managers run the hospital, recruiting, training and retaining staff from many disciplines, optimising use of operating theatres, beds and clinics, managing IT systems and planning major rebuilds and refurbishments, while wards remain open twenty-four hours a day, seven days a week.

It is not just in hospitals that systems have become more complex. The days when general practitioners operated from privately owned premises with a minimum of support staff, subscribed to a single medical journal, phoned a specialist when they needed advice and did about an hour's paperwork a week are long gone (Plsek and Greenhalgh 2001: 625). GPs now work in large multidisciplinary teams and partnerships that are themselves linked into yet larger organisational networks (see Chapter 3). They are no longer autonomous decision-makers when it comes to practice management.

Given the complexity of this extraordinary tapestry of interwoven activities, it is perhaps not surprising that care delivery is not always perfect – whether at Great Ormond Street, the Albion, St Michael's or in any other hospital or health-care setting. Of course, we should not lose sight of the fact that, on the whole, the important aspects of Daniel's early care went very well. His bowel obstruction was diagnosed promptly, he was transferred rapidly to a specialist centre and his operation was successful. The clinical staff knew that this kind of bowel obstruction is one way in which cystic fibrosis can declare itself, so they had done all the necessary tests to confirm or refute this – although they had not discussed the possibility with his parents.

But for Susan some points in the journey leading up to the meeting with Dr Hill will be etched on her memory forever – as will the meeting itself. For example: the long ambulance ride to the Albion, not understanding why Daniel had to be transferred because the doctor at St Michael's was bleeped away before he could finish his explanation;

the period of anxiety and uncertainty in the weeks before his follow-up appointment when she had no point of contact at the Albion and didn't know who else to talk to; and the long wait in Outpatients as Dr Hill's appointments slipped progressively more and more behind schedule. Patients appreciate the expertise of the clinicians who care for them, but it is often the system glitches rather than their actual clinical management that leave them feeling frustrated, angry and sometimes moved to make a complaint.

Do these things really matter? One could argue that these are the soft edges of health care; that the heroic, lifesaving aspects are the only important facets, and optimising the rest of the patient experience is a luxury that the NHS can ill afford. In reality, any one who has lived for weeks or even months with uncertainty, who has suffered delayed or missed appointments, who has not been given the information they need for reassurance, will know that these things matter a great deal. They are the signs of a vulnerable organisational system and do not inspire confidence in the quality of that system's clinical care.

Of course, it is easy to see patients as the main 'victims' of stretched or faulty systems, but that is an oversimplification. Sebastian Hill was also feeling 'out of control'. From his perspective, he'd been let down by the specialist nurse who should have been there to help him discuss the diagnosis of cystic fibrosis with the Johnsons. The clinic was overbooked, the results he needed weren't available, the interpreter was late, and while he was sure there were some patient leaflets about cystic fibrosis somewhere in the department, he didn't have time to look for them. It is easy to lay the blame at his feet. After all, surely he should have called his consultant when he had a niggling doubt that this was not a consultation that he should have handled alone? But it is also important to ask whether his training should have equipped him to deal more effectively with the situation in which he found himself.

From 'machines' to 'complex adaptive systems'

Why does so much of the NHS appear to be caught in a web of increasing stress and complexity, and what can be done about it?

In the early 1900s, much of our understanding about running organisations came from industry and factory management (NHS Confederation 2001a). The entire factory would function like a well-oiled machine with very simple rules about the exact numbers of staff and components needed to generate anything from car parts to condoms. Each part of the organisation could be given very precise directions, and the outputs were entirely predictable.

> The laws of physics may perfectly predict how one gas particle interacts with another gas particle, but it is impossible to use these laws to forecast with perfect accuracy what the weather will be like tomorrow.
>
> (Papadopoulos et al. 2001: 613)

GOSH in 1852 may have followed these simple rules under the watchful eye of that first matron. GOSH more than 150 years later does not – and nor does the rest of the health-care system. We now understand that hospitals and health-care networks function as 'complex adaptive systems'. This means that each part of each organisation has a life of its own, with some freedom to act independently. If a new directive or plan is put forward, not only will each unit within the system interpret and implement it slightly differently, but when all these units interact with each other, the results may be radically different from those that were intended or expected. Science writer Richard Dawkins has described this as the difference between launching a bird and launching a rock (NHS Confederation 2001a). Careful calculation will tell us something about the trajectory and landing place of the rock, but the bird is a different matter.

For example, suppose a surgical unit has a certain number of consultants and a long waiting list. The obvious plan might be to employ another consultant. One consequence of this is that local GPs, knowing there is a new consultant, may lower their threshold for making referrals. At the same time, the other consultants may feel able to spend more time with each patient in clinic. The result is that the waiting time to see a consultant could go up. Worse still, if the new consultant post is not matched by extra theatre staff, extra X-ray facilities, more catering staff, more beds and so on, bottlenecks will build up elsewhere in the system, and the problems will become even worse (Papadopoulos et al. 2001: 613). Simplistic solutions do not work, because trying to fix just one part of a system can have all sorts of consequences in other parts of the system. Then, as new problems creep into the system, clinicians and managers create their own new rules to set it on track again – and suddenly there is more bureaucracy, more complexity. Meanwhile, everyone is puzzled about why the talented new consultant has done nothing to reduce the length of the waiting list. Shortage of staff and resources is an important element of the problem, and this will be revisited in Chapter 4. But launching a bird rather than a rock can have all sorts of quite unexpected consequences that have little to do with resources and much to do with the overall system.

The Government, finding itself in the bird-launching rather than the rock-throwing business, faces a difficult dilemma. On the one hand, it has committed billions of pounds to improving the systems and performance of the NHS. This gives a powerful political imperative to specify rules, targets and outcomes to justify the investment and demonstrate its effectiveness. On the other hand, the tighter the rules and targets, the greater the danger of stifling the creativity that is essential to the development and improvement of the system and of producing unintended results. Whilst targets remain a central part of the performance-management philosophy, it is equally essential to look at systems as living, dynamic organisms and to harness their powers of independent flight.

Surviving and harnessing complex systems

There are several possible approaches to untangling complex systems. The most politically obvious is to stand outside the system and to plan overarching NHS-wide strategies and targets to try to change things inside. The 'outside–in' approach, which stems from the factory and widget philosophy, is useful up to a point but, for the reasons given above, it ultimately becomes counterproductive, and alternative strategies need to be brought in. The other side of the coin is to start inside the system – with the patient's experience of what went wrong – and to use that experience to take an 'inside-out' approach to problem solving.

Starting with the patient

When Susan and Matthew left the Outpatient Department after their appointment with Dr Hill, the system had let them down at several steps along the road and had left them in a state of grief and distress. The Patient Advice and Liaison Service (PALS) is an important source of help for patients and families such as the Johnsons. Established in 2002, PALSs have been set up in hospitals across the country to provide on-the-spot help for patients, families and carers in all kinds of circumstances, acting as gateways to independent advice and advocacy and providing information about available services.

If Susan had known about them when she wanted help, they could have put her in touch with the right people, locally or at the Albion. Susan's situation was rather unusual, because problems with young babies are most often picked up by health visitors who, after the early days of midwife support are over, become key points of contact for families with children up to the age of five. But where, as in Daniel's case, a baby goes direct to a specialist centre rather than coming home, there is always a danger that discharge letters will not reach the GP or the health visitor before their first visit. In this situation, the PALS team would not have replaced existing services or processes that should have been in place. But they would have been able to bridge the gap, to make the right connections and to identify the holes that families like the Johnsons can fall into.

PALS teams are important because their *raison d'être* is to make things better for individual patients. But they are also catalysts for change and improvement. They are the eyes and ears of the hospital, helping staff to identify system glitches. The Snakes and Ladders project started at GOSH at around the same time that the PALS team was established. Having the PALS team on the project-steering group was invaluable. It meant that as soon as families brought problems to them, we could rapidly dramatise them on stage (in an anonymous way), bring them to the attention of staff and look for solutions.

Planning the system nationally

Not all problems are amenable to local solutions. Sebastian Hill's appointments were running late because a series of circumstances had conspired against him. The clinic was overbooked, notes and results had gone missing and the nurse specialist was off sick. Some large-scale nationally developed improvements to the system and infrastructure may have helped him.

For example, a frequent barrier to running clinics efficiently is the number of patients who 'do not attend' (termed DNAs). Clinic receptionists try to manage this by overbooking clinics, on the basis that there will be a regular percentage of DNAs. But there is always the risk that on some days most patients will attend and wait for an unacceptable length of time, becoming increasingly stressed and anxious, as was the case for Susan and Matthew. To give some perspective on the problem, in England in 2000/1, more than 1.5 million patients failed to attend a first outpatient appointment, and more than 4 million failed to attend subsequent ones (Managing DNAs 2003). Each DNA costs the NHS at least 50 pounds. This totals about 275 million pounds a year, complicates waiting-list management and leaves some patients without treatment.

> Considering the strain the NHS is under to meet demand, the cost of missed appointments can be ill afforded. At the end of the day each missed appointment means more time waiting in the surgery.
>
> (Dr Simon Fradd, Chairman, Doctor Patient Partnership, Public Fails to Cancel Appointments 1999)

A national programme has now been set in place to tackle this problem through a partnership approach with patients. By giving patients choice about when they attend clinics, and by negotiating an appointment slot, it is anticipated that attendance will be substantially improved. Where the new system has been piloted, DNA rates have fallen and this has had a knock-on effect of reducing waiting times to first appointments.

It seems extraordinary that missing results, X-ray and patient records still beset clinicians on a daily basis. Whilst electronic booking is now in sight, the progress of the electronic patient record is still patchy. X-rays and laboratory results are available electronically in a growing number of hospitals, but patients still have bulky and incomplete notes, with poorly filed information. GP surgeries have had both electronic prescribing and electronic patient records in place for many years, but it seems that hospital notes and handwritten drug charts will be with us for some time. This inevitably means that space has to be found for storage, expensive archiving systems have to be maintained and, at the most frustrating level, staff have to be employed to tramp round doctors' offices, outpatient departments and clinic rooms, trying to find case notes that are not where they are supposed to be.

The pot of gold at the end of the rainbow is the National Programme for Information Technology – a 6.2 billion pound project which promises to create a basic health record for all 50 million patients and to connect more than 30,000 GPs and 270 acute, community and mental-health trusts in a secure system (Humber 2004: 1145). Can such an ambitious project succeed? Thus far, it has won the hearts and minds of senior politicians and Department of Health leaders, but has yet to engage health-care professionals and the public.

In truth we should not be asking whether this project will succeed, but rather whether we can possibly afford to let it fail. The significance of poor information management goes beyond waiting times in Outpatients. The report into the tragic death of Victoria Climbié (Laming 2003) highlighted the contribution made by poor and fragmented case records and recommended a single set of notes for each patient on any one site. The entire NHS reform programme, the drive for better access and choice and the need to reduce clinical errors are all dependent on a revolution in information and communications technology.

Managing the system locally

National booking systems and electronic records require central coordination. There is no point in individual hospitals all inventing the wheel in isolation and developing systems that won't 'talk to each other'. However, the management and 'ironing-out' of local systems and processes has to rest with local teams.

Banner headlines frequently condemn the 'soaring numbers of managers' in the NHS, when the perception is that we need more clinicians. There is a naivety to this mantra. We do, of course, need more clinicians. But it is not possible to have an accountable health service with streamlined patient access without the management infrastructure to support it. The role of NHS managers stretches from mundane but crucially important practicalities such as making sure notes are available in clinic, to tackling a recruitment programme for the country's largest employer, administering a budget of over 60 billion pounds and juggling limited staff and resources. Indeed, the public would be far more alarmed if trained clinical staff were deployed to manage outpatient departments and to review booking systems.

The debate on NHS reform is dogged by the accusation that money is being wasted on an army of managers and administrators. The accusation that there are 'more bureaucrats than beds' has become a convenient soundbite, endlessly repeated by those who believe the current reforms are making little impact.
(NHS Confederation 2004: 1)

For example, the perverse mystery of how clinical notes and X-rays vanish at the very time they are most needed is not one that requires investigative genius. Every hospital has sound policies and procedures about filling in tracer cards, keeping notes in subscribed areas and not taking them off-site. But clinical staff break these rules – not because they are being obstructive, but because they are busy, they just want to get an urgent letter written for their patient, and they have every intention of returning the notes 'in a few minutes'. So service managers spend a great deal of time auditing the number of missing notes, finding new ways to communicate with clinicians, trying to make the system more flexible and practical, and auditing again.

Not only are managers themselves essential to delivery of service but so too is the management perspective. Clinicians are professionally driven to focus on the patient in the bed in front of them, but managers must focus equally on all the patients not yet in the bed or in the clinic and on the most efficient way to get them there.

> If managers suddenly became preoccupied with the needs of an individual patient, irrespective of the consequences for others or for their budget, then the health system would collapse. If doctors decided that their principal concern was to ensure the smooth running of the system and the delivery of policy irrespective of the consequences for the patient in front of them, then both the quality of care and public support would collapse. Doctors worry about patient outcomes. Managers worry about patient experience (which includes outcomes, but only as part of a mix to be met out of finite resources). Patients are, again, best served by a tension between the two.
>
> (Edwards et al. 2003: 609)

Combining national guidance and local creativity

Is it possible to have accountability, adherence to nationally agreed targets and the freedom to adapt local systems so that they deliver the best care for patients – or does this impossible tension mean that the whole system will collapse in a complex mess? An example will illustrate the answer: for a patient having a heart attack, survival is improved if a clot-dissolving drug is injected within an hour of the pain starting. This is called thrombolysis therapy. One could micro-manage the whole system and say that the ambulance had to arrive within fifteen minutes of a call from a patient with chest pain, that the door-to-needle time in the acute hospital had to be no more than thirty minutes, and so on. Then each team within the process would act independently of each other, working on their own tiny part of the process. The ambulance service and the A&E department might compete for money, because both might think they needed more staff to meet their 'thrombolysis target'. The alternative is to provide national guidance about what is needed and then to ask the ambulance service, the GPs and the acute trusts to work out how to tackle the problem in their area together. Rather than employing more ambulance drivers, the solution may be better education of patients so that they call an ambulance sooner, or removal of some road humps that are slowing down traffic. In this scenario, everyone may perform better if given a minimum specification – a set of guiding principles – rather than a series of targets (NHS Confederation 2001a). Direction and flexibility need to be combined.

Box 2.1 Learning points for clinicians and patients: complex systems

- System failings, such as overbooked clinics, long waits and missing notes can be as distressing for patients as a clinical error.
- Some problems require nationally led changes in policy and major changes to the infrastructure. Other problems can be dealt with by local creativity and ownership.
- Everyone has responsibility for making local systems work, both staff and patients.
- For many aspects of the care process, guidance and direction-setting work better than strict targets.
- Information from individual patients can be invaluable in spotting and solving problems in the system.
- Chapter 4 will give more information about how both staff and patients can get involved in system improvement.

THE SOCIETAL CONTEXT: CULTURAL BACKDROP

> Much of the misunderstanding in communication comes from assuming that the other person understands what you are saying. However, in many cases, factors such as emotions and differences in cultural background and education can blur the message as it passes from 'giver' to 'receiver.'
>
> (Health Canada 2001: 11)

One of the 'external' factors described in Chapter 1 of this book – the factors that exist independently of the hospital procedures or the specifics of the consultation itself – is the cultural and belief system that all parties bring with them to the hospital, the prior experience that shapes their response to illness and their expectations of their treatment.

An advertisement for a well-known bank highlights the importance of 'local knowledge'. A man is shown putting his feet up, usually synonymous with relaxation. But we are told that to do this in Thailand, to show the soles of your feet, is gravely offensive. Cecil Helman has written extensively on the subject of cultural response to health and illness. He defines culture as follows:

> Culture is the set of guidelines (both explicit and implicit) which individuals inherit as members of a particular society, and which tell them how to view the world, how to experience it *emotionally*, how to *behave* in it in relation to other people, to supernatural forces or gods, and to the natural environment. To some extent, culture can be seen as an inherited 'lens' through which people perceive and understand the world that they inhabit . . .
>
> (Helman 2003: 2)

Susan and Matthew are an English-speaking Caucasian couple from similar cultural, educational and social backgrounds – and yet they bring such different experiences and personalities with them that it would be hard to pitch information in a way that would suit both. If one or both of them was from a different continent or culture, or had a very different belief system about the origins and management of illness, the consultation would have been even more fraught than it already was.

Our cultural and societal background influences our most basic understanding of what illness is and how to respond to it. Cassell (1976) explains that the word 'illness' stands for 'what the patient feels when he goes to the doctor', whilst 'disease' is 'what he has on the way home from the doctor's office'. In Western society, medicine is based on scientific rationality, a belief system in which all assumptions and hypotheses must be capable of being tested and verified under objective, empirical and controlled conditions. Lay theories of illness causation are much broader and are discussed in detail by Helman (2003), in his excellent book *Culture Health and Illness*.

As a broad generalisation, in industrialised societies lay explanations of illness tend to focus on either the individual patient or on the environment. Patient-focused explanations include diet, hygiene, lifestyle, relationships and so on. These explanations are often tied into a level of blame or guilt; for example, about eating the wrong foods, not taking enough exercise, being sexually promiscuous or not taking care of oneself. Environmental explanations are in the ascendancy and include food additives, mobile-phone masts, pollutants and genetically modified foods. In this case, the perceived blame is external to the patient and is possibly focused on the administration or government.

In non-industrialised societies, explanations can be very different and may be focused in the social or the supernatural world. Social causes of illness are most often based on interpersonal malevolence: witchcraft, voodoo, hexes and the evil eye are all examples of this. When supernatural forces – gods or spirits – result in illness, this is sometimes seen as a result of the sins or failures of the sufferer, but sometimes also due to the capriciousness of the gods and hence unrelated to any actions on the part of the victim. Possession is another common theme and can again be related to immoral or blasphemous behaviour, with illness being the resulting punishment. Finally, 'acts of God', karma, fate or 'the stars' cross many societal boundaries as a rationalisation of illness.

Sebastian's belief in a genetic mutation as the cause of Daniel's illness is the only one that he truly entertains. While at a cognitive level he may be aware of other belief systems, he will see them as just that: belief systems that do not hold any fundamental truth for him.

Thus, he will frame his explanation of the illness in his own terms, as well as the ways in which it should be managed. Equally, his cultural and belief system will colour his terminology, the way in which he expects the Johnsons to react and his perception of 'normal' distress behaviours.

Davis (2003) recently highlighted the complexity of cultural and linguistic differences and the risk of misunderstandings in relation to the Chinese community in the English-speaking world. The Chinese view that 'Shameful business should not be discussed outside the family' may make it particularly difficult for health professionals to gather from and discuss information with patients or families. Interpreters need to be very clear about their duty of confidentiality, which should be overtly stated in front of the family. Another difference that can lead to misunderstandings concerns the degree of physical contact between parents and children. The Chinese encourage it far less than many other cultures, and professionals have interpreted this as emotional coldness: 'In an hour, that family never once comforted their children.' The issues raised are not unique to this group and illustrate wider challenges.

This vast array of cultural differences need to be borne in mind not just when giving a diagnosis, but also when discussing treatment options, considering issues of confidentiality, managing pain relief, discussing end-of-life decisions and, indeed, at every stage in the patient–clinician relationship. A full discussion of the issues is outside the scope of this book, but the interested reader may gain further insights from Cecil Helman's book or related texts.

AT THE FRONT LINE: THE CONSULTATION

With all these issues in mind, we are finally at the stage of being able to take a constructive view of what happened in the meeting between Sebastian and the Johnsons and of how it might have been different if he had been able to 'rewind' and start again.

Preparation

The best Sebastian had managed to do by way of preparation in our scenario was to try and get himself to the clinic and to take a few deep breaths and straighten his tie before seeing the Johnsons. He was ill prepared before he even opened the door in trying to get things right. None the less, there are always opportunities to do better, and the following outlines some of the important principles to consider when breaking bad news or facing difficult conversations with patients:

Make sure you are the right person to be delivering the news

In our scenario, Sebastian probably wasn't the right person but was precipitated into the role by circumstances. He could, and should, have asked his consultant to help him, but that is easily said with hindsight. In other settings – for example, had Daniel still been an inpatient – there would have been more time to talk the situation through with his consultant. This would have allowed the consultant to judge whether Sebastian was the best person to talk to the Johnsons and also to rehearse with him the outline of the consultation and the key points to cover.

Two practicalities determine whether a clinician is in a good position to break bad news to patients: training and experience. Doctors in training tend to worry a great deal about whether they will miss an important clinical sign, or make a prescription error or a mistake during an operation. In fact, poor communication is far more likely to culminate in a complaint or clinical problem. For example, in 2000–1 there were 140,000 formal complaints about NHS services. Of the 95,000 complaints about hospital services, attitudes of staff (13 per cent) and communication and information to patients (9 per cent) were among the top four categories of complaint (Department of Health 2003a). In recognition of this issue, the Department of Health is in the throes of radically revising the training of junior doctors to ensure that they receive 'generic skills training' during their first two years in practice. This will encompass many different facets including effective relationships with patients, communication skills and working in teams.

Make sure you have the right information

In this instance, having the 'right information' was not just about having Daniel's records and results to hand. It certainly should have included getting his name right, an apparently crass, but not infrequent mistake made by health-care workers under stress or pressure.

Outside of these rather obvious principles, Sebastian needed to have information about cystic fibrosis for both himself and for the Johnsons. For clinicians, the increasing availability of evidence-based information on-line has had a transformational effect on the way we practise medicine. Many clinicians have become so distracted by focusing on the negative aspects of the Internet that they have overlooked the benefits it provides, which include a broad array of information, albeit of varying quality, medical on-line support groups and the opportunity to conduct e-based research (Ferguson and Frydman 2004: 1148).

Box 2.2 Learning points for clinicians: accessing information

- Visit the National Electronic Library for Health at <http://www.nelh.nhs.uk> where you will be able to access the Cochrane database and a wide range of other electronic resources.
- Ask your hospital librarian for an Athens account, which will allow you to access a wider range of electronic literature.
- If possible, enrol on a course on evidence-based practice. This will help you to evaluate the literature much more effectively.
- Bear in mind that despite your own natural anxiety about the quality of information on the Internet, reports of patients coming to harm as the result of on-line advice are rare, whereas accounts of those who obtained better care are common.

(Ferguson and Frydman 2004: 1148)

Ideally, Sebastian also needed to be able to give or at least point the Johnsons to the wide range of patient leaflets and literature that cover the vast majority of common illnesses – as well as many very rare conditions. He should also have been able to provide them with details of relevant self-help groups, which are a major source of mutual support. Several learning points emerge when considering sources of information:

Box 2.3 Learning points for patients: accessing information

- When you receive a new diagnosis, ask the doctor about any resources available for patients – either written or on-line.
- If you feel ready to do so, ask about self-help groups or, if you want a more personal first approach, you may want to ask the clinician if they can put you in touch with another patient with the same condition.
- The Internet can be an excellent source of information. However, seeing information in print (or pixels!) gives it a ring of truth; do bear in mind that the source of the information is important and that the quality of information will vary widely, so try and verify what you read.
- If you bring information from the web to show to your doctor for advice, do not be surprised if he or she has not seen it before. The pace at which information burgeons on the web is astounding, so your clinician may not be able to give you an instant response to your query about it.

Make sure the environment and timing is right

Circumstances sometimes result in patients being given difficult diagnoses in hospital corridors, on the end of a phone, or in the middle of a busy ward. At times this is unavoidable. Wherever possible, however, it is important to find a quiet room, to switch off bleeps and mobile phones (and that applies to patients as well as doctors) and to avoid interruptions.

If you have a choice about timing, try to schedule the meeting early in the day so that families do not have to wait, worrying, before the meeting, or being left to cope with bad news alone at night. Set against that, don't schedule a difficult meeting if you will have insufficient time to spend with the family.

Make sure the right people are there

> It's vital to have someone else there, in the room, to pick up the pieces. A consultant in a busy clinic simply can't spend all day clarifying facts or telling parents about support organizations. There may be two or three other families waiting, about to go through a similar trauma. But just as much as the doctor may not have time, parents or patients will almost certainly need it.
>
> (Bea Teuten, Family Advocate, PALS, GOSH)

Bea Teuten, who leads the PALS service at GOSH has a daughter with complex, multiple health problems. As a parent, she has become familiar with receiving bad news. As a professional, she often has to cope with the emotional fallout when it is broken badly.

Recalling her own experiences, she describes the importance of having a third party, such as a clinical nurse specialist, present at meetings where news is shared. These nurses have an increasingly important role to play in the NHS, developing expertise in specific areas and often being vital sources of information and support for people with both common or rare conditions.

This is another reason why it is so important for doctors, whenever possible, to talk to patients and families with a colleague present, usually a member of nursing staff. It leaves a second person available to continue the conversation if the doctor is called away and helps ensure that other staff, such as the nursing team, know what has been said and can follow up on any queries. Whilst the clinical nurse specialist who should have been there with Sebastian was off sick, and he'd run shy of asking his consultant, he could have asked one of the other nurses in the outpatient clinic to join him.

As well as ensuring that a second professional is present, it is also important to try and ensure that the patient is not alone. When giving a diagnosis about a child, it is important to try and have both parents present, although family breakdowns may mean that this is not always possible. It may also be appropriate for the child to be present; with a younger child it is always worth checking out parental views on this in advance. For adults, another family member or a friend is just as important. Sometimes a friend can help by writing down what the doctor says at a time when the patient is finding the information difficult to absorb.

If you are using a professional interpreter, make sure you have obtained family consent. Also ensure that the family knows that the interpreter understands confidentiality. Language Line (0800 169 2879) is the service used by most UK hospitals.

The beginning of the consultation

The preliminaries

The first few moments of a consultation can set the scene for the next half hour. When things get off on the wrong footing, it is sometimes almost impossible to recover. In our scenario, Sebastian should have introduced himself and apologised for keeping the Johnsons waiting – regardless of whether or not he was feeling aggrieved that the delay was not his fault. Establishing rapport is critically important, and much of Sebastian's discomfort and subsequent panic may have been because he had not made a connection with the family.

Check out prior knowledge

Sebastian launched into his explanation of cystic fibrosis without any knowledge of what the words meant to Susan and Matthew. As it happened, they had very little meaning for Matthew, but for Susan they conjured up an image of a frail and sickly schoolmate who had died prematurely. Once that image had leapt into her mind, it was impossible for her to focus on anything Sebastian said thereafter. If he had known anything about her preconceptions about the illness, he would have been able to explore them with her, to explain the differences in treatment since she was a child, to free her up to ask more questions and maybe to lessen slightly the immediate trauma. It is at this point that cultural differences in perceptions of the illness can be uncovered.

The middle of the consultation

The first thing to understand about the middle of the consultation is that the patient may remember very little of what is said. This is a normal reaction, and is not just about unfamiliarity with the concepts. Health-care professionals have exactly the same problem when they themselves are patients.

Box 2.4 Learning points for clinicians: checking out prior knowledge

The following open-ended questions show how Sebastian could have initiated the consultation in order to elicit Susan's concerns and prior beliefs:

- How has Daniel been?
- Was there anything you wanted to discuss about his progress since he left hospital?
- Have you come with some questions you wanted to ask me?

Once Susan has raised concerns, he could follow up with:

- Have you had any thoughts yourself about why Daniel has not been gaining weight?

Susan has had thoughts about this. The possibility of cystic fibrosis was raised in her mind on the ward, and she may already have been on the Internet and found out that this is a strong possibility. Once the words 'cystic fibrosis' have been used for the first time, whether by Susan or Sebastian, he could ask:

- Cystic fibrosis means many different things to different people. Have you heard of it before?
- What do you already know about the condition?

Box 2.5 Learning points for patients: preparing for a consultation

- If you are expecting to receive an important diagnosis, try and take someone with who can act as a 'second pair of ears'.
- Write down a list of questions that you would like to cover before the consultation – and don't be afraid to take them out and work through them with the clinician.
- Don't be afraid to mention worries that you may have about the problem. You may think they are 'silly' or unfounded, but rest assured that many previous patients will have had the same thoughts or concerns.

Try and make the information as manageable as possible

The following tips outline how to try and maximise the patient's ability to absorb what has been said:

Box 2.6 Learning points for clinicians: the middle of the consultation

- Try and signpost what you are going to say. For example, 'There are three important things I am going to cover. First I want to explain . . . now we'll move on to . . .'.
- Keep language simple, and avoid jargon.
- Speak slowly and use repetition.
- Use visual supports – models or diagrams – where appropriate.
- Check what the patient has understood of what you have said, and give frequent chances to ask questions or contribute their own thoughts.
- Relate your explanation to what the patient has already told you about their concepts or understanding of the condition.
- Where appropriate, back up what you have said with written information.

(Adapted from Kurtz and Silverman 1996: 83)

Avoid premature reassurance

Giving premature reassurance is an intensely human reaction. We all do it all the time. Our first response to the friend who says they are afraid they might fail their impending exam is inevitably, 'Don't worry, you'll be fine.' As clinicians, we certainly do it during consultations:

'I don't know how I'm going to cope.'
'Don't worry, you'll be fine.'

'But he's so vulnerable.'
'Oh, I'm sure he's tougher than you think.'

'Supposing I'm the one in a 1,000 people who doesn't survive this operation?'
'Don't worry, I'm sure you won't be.'

By using 'safe' responses like these, even very senior clinicians can fall into the trap of blocking cues and stopping people from talking about their fears and worries, when they may desperately need to do so. Practising simple skills such as asking an open question to enable the patient to share feelings (as opposed to a closed or leading question whereby the patient will only give the answer expected by the doctor) can transform an encounter. If Sebastian had been able to do this, he would have been able to respond to and explore the Johnsons' real concerns and worries rather than reinforcing his own assumptions and then struggling to decide 'what to say'.

Maguire and Pitceathly (2002: 697) explain how getting this right not only improves the outcome for patients, but actually improves the well-being of the doctor imparting the news. Whilst it is not always possible to avoid this behaviour, it is possible to recognise it for what it is and to make a mental note to come back later and explore the issues, when maybe the time pressures are not so great.

It is important to cover 'the worst' at the first interview, acknowledging the enormity of it all. You may lose families' trust if you backtrack later because you gave false reassurance or hope at the outset.

The end of the consultation

Sometimes the relief of getting a piece of news across successfully is so great that the end of the consultation slips away without reaching a proper conclusion. There are two important aspects to closing the consultation.

Agree a plan

Agreeing a management plan actually means a negotiated agreement with the patient, rather than a prescriptive decision by the clinician. Arriving at an agreed plan is not always straightforward and is discussed in much more detail in later chapters. As part of the planning process, it is essential that the patient knows when they will next be seen, by whom and who they can contact in the interim if they have concerns. However bad the situation, end with a positive plan of support.

Record what has been said and agreed in the notes

Once again, this may sound like a statement of the obvious, but clinicians are very likely to note that a diagnosis was given without noting any of the specifics about patient concerns, the precise words that were used, the topics that there was not time to cover and so on. This is equally important to jog the memory of the same clinician if they see the patient on the next visit or to prompt other people who may pick up subsequent questions or problems.

Tell patients and families when they will receive letters after meetings and, with older children, agree when letters will be shared with parents and when sent exclusively to them.

And afterwards

Patients and families may want to meet up with other people who have had a similar illness or diagnosis. Voluntary sector organisations have a crucial role to play, and many are very active in providing support networks and even attending outpatient clinics to support new patients. For example, Contact a Family (0808 808 3555, <http://www.cafmily.org.uk>) is an excellent national charity dedicated to helping families who care for children with any disability or special need. It is important for both patients and clinicians to be aware of this kind of resource, but to remember that individuals will vary a great deal in terms of if and when they might want to access self-help groups.

At the end of the day

'At the moment, I'm beginning to feel like I'm never going to make a good clinician or an academic,' Sebastian said to Dr Val Sharpe, ten minutes into his appraisal meeting in her office.

It was a week after Sebastian's meeting with the Johnsons, and he had not been looking forward to spending an hour talking to his consultant about where his career was going and what he needed to learn during his year at the Albion.

To a large extent, he realised that he was probably overreacting. It was just that he had invested so much in his plan to become a specialist in respiratory paediatrics, had been elated when he got this job; and now suddenly everything seemed to be going horribly wrong. It wasn't just the failure to get his research project funded; in fact, over the past few months, his interest in the clinical side of paediatrics had become more important to him than pursuing an academic career – and maybe that was why he wasn't entirely focused when he wrote the funding application. It was more a case that two weeks into the job he was feeling rather inept and deskilled. Everyone seemed to know more than him. The nurses on the ward, the physiotherapist, even the other junior doctors. The episode with the Johnsons had been just one of a series of events where he had got things wrong or where he had to ask for help, and he had come to the conclusion that Dr Sharpe had probably already written him off as an idiot. It was a novel experience for someone who had always got what he wanted with minimal effort.

'I mean, just last week, there was that meeting with the Johnsons. I know you've heard about it already, because they phoned the ward in such a state the next day. I realise that I shouldn't have ploughed into the consultation by myself, but I did think I might have managed it better than a first-year medical student. After all, it's not as if I don't have quite a lot of experience of breaking bad news to parents from my previous jobs . . .'

He paused for a moment, but before Dr Sharpe was able to get a word in, he rushed on through his stream of self-castigation.

'I suppose the thing I wasn't prepared for was their total silence when I told them the diagnosis. Maybe if I'd given them a bit more time to frame their thoughts and ask some questions, it would have been OK. But I just felt like I had to fill the silence, so I started rambling on in completely incomprehensible jargon, and they just kept sitting there looking at me blankly. I know I wasn't exactly in great form that day, but still . . . how can anyone manage a consultation that badly after being qualified for seven years?'

Dimly aware that he was doing exactly the same thing now – rambling on without giving his listener a chance to respond – he finally tailed into silence.

'Actually, I still have consultations that go badly after being qualified for nearly twenty years,' Dr Sharpe said wryly. 'That's just life. The difference is, I'm just better at minimising the bad consultations, blocking out the other things that are on my mind and using a wider range of strategies to maintain an open dialogue with families.'

Watching the relief spread over Sebastian's face, she decided it was safe to tackle the broader problem that she'd discussed the previous day with the ward sister.

'Look Sebastian, you are right. I have had some feedback from the nurses on Starlight ward because they can see you're struggling to settle in. I think maybe you've just had so much invested in this job that you're trying too hard. You don't have to come in knowing everything about respiratory paediatrics. That's what you're here to learn. It is alright to ask; that's what working in a team is about. And it is alright that the nurses know more than you. Some of them have been here for years. When I started working here, I was pretty convinced that even the cleaner seemed to know more about the running of the unit than I did – and I mean that literally; she'd been here eight years at the time.'

Sebastian smiled for the first time since coming into the room. 'Hmm, maybe I have been overreacting a bit,' he said. 'Bit of a crisis of confidence.'

Dr Sharpe had been here on several occasions with new junior doctors, and she felt relatively confident that this one was going to be alright. He wasn't one of the ones that bothered her; she could deal fairly easily with the ones who magnified their failings and took a while to find their feet. It was the ones who did not seem to have any insight that she really lost sleep about. She'd had one such only six months previously. A girl who was exceptionally bright, knew all the right answers and could quote the latest research, but who was persistently rude to the nurses, upset the patients and often left work early, after dumping unfinished tasks on her colleagues. Despite some pretty frank feedback she had remained convinced that she was performing well and managed to reframe situations so that any problems that occurred were somehow down to someone else. Dr Sharpe had an uncomfortable feeling that she was going to be just as much trouble in her next job. She couldn't help wondering whether the selection criteria for medical school were still weighted too heavily in favour of exam results rather than appropriate temperament and personality – but how to get that right?

UNRESOLVED QUESTIONS: INSIGHT AND PERFORMANCE

> The story of the paediatric cardiac surgical services in Bristol is not an account of bad people. Nor is it an account of people who did not care, nor of people who wilfully harm patients. It is an account of people who cared greatly about human suffering, and were dedicated and well motivated. Sadly, some lacked insight and their behaviour was flawed. Many failed to communicate with each other, and to work together effectively for the interests of their patients. There was a lack of leadership, and of team-work.
>
> (Bristol Royal Infirmary Inquiry 2001: 1)

The above is one of the most oft-quoted extracts from the independent inquiry into paediatric cardiac surgery in Bristol. Since that time, much has been done to address the many systemic shortcomings that allowed the crisis to occur. Among other changes, appraisal and revalidation for consultant staff has been established by the General Medical Council (GMC).

Appraisal is not a novel concept for the medical profession; it has been in place for doctors in training since the late 1990s, earlier and in general than in hospital practice. By contrast, the current generation of consultants has not previously been appraised. What is also new is the sense that accountability and teamwork can and must replace the traditional autonomy and independent practice that has characterised the consultant role. These values must be developed throughout the training programme, starting at medical school and must be reinforced through the junior training years. Val Sharpe's meeting with Sebastian Hill was an example of the importance of this process in action.

On a positive note, public trust in doctors has remained high, despite the run of high-profile medical scandals – Shipman, Ledward, Bristol, Alder Hay and Meadows. By 2004, doctors were still continuing to come out top in MORI's annual poll of the most trusted professionals or occupational groups (British Medical Association and MORI 2004). Ninety-two per cent of the public said that they trusted doctors, compared with 89 per cent for teachers, 75 per cent for judges and priests, 22 per cent for politicians and 20 per cent for journalists. In fact, trust in the medical profession has risen steadily from 82 per cent in 1983 to 92 per cent in 2004. This suggests that the public is able to separate the information about extreme cases from their more experiential impressions, based on personal health-care encounters, and this is discussed more fully in Chapter 3. These findings may also reflect a greater sophistication in the public's understanding and expectation of the medical role. Within the more paternalistic model of previous years, it was often seen as appropriate that doctors did not always tell the truth and that this was justified by the need to spare patients' fears and anxieties, for example in relation to terminal illness. Currently there is rightly an expectation of full information sharing (see Chapters 6 and 7).

Comforting as the MORI data may be for the medical profession, there is no room for complacency. Events of the past few years have highlighted the need to provide the public with better protection – not just from the one in a million Shipmans, but from poorly performing doctors more generally. The links between safeguards around professional performance, patient safety, patient involvement, inspection and review were outlined in a document called *A Commitment to Quality, A Quest for Excellence* (Department of Health 2001a). The document represents a sign-up between the Government, the NHS and the medical profession. It sets out expectations on the public and the media, as well as on clinicians and the Department of Health, in terms of their responsibilities to the NHS. There is a commitment to delivering high-quality health-care delivery alongside an acknowledgement that poor performance is the province of the few.

Sir Donald Irvine (President of the GMC, 1995–2002) recently retold the Bristol story in his book *The Doctor's Tale: Professionalism and Public Trust* (Irvine 2003). It is a book that describes the changing relationship between the public and their doctors. In subsequent lectures and papers, he has gone on to discuss the further steps that the profession needs to take in order to redefine that relationship in a way that is compatible with the twenty-first-century values and

Matters came to a head with the tragedy in paediatric cardiac surgery at Bristol. Laid bare were doctors' collective attitude towards audit, teamwork, whistleblowing, consent to treatment and complaints about poor practice that evoked words such as reactive, protective and inward-looking.

(Irvine 2004: 271)

expectations. There are two key issues. The first is the need to replace paternalism with shared responsibility and decision-making, and this will be elaborated in Chapters 6 and 7. The second is the need to ensure that the profession is properly regulated.

The performance-management framework for doctors has undergone transformational change since Bristol, but a recent editorial in the *British Medical Journal* (Smith 2005: 1) warns that those changes may be too little, too late. Dame Janet Smith DBE, the High Court judge who chaired the independent public inquiry into the Shipman case, released her fifth report in December 2004 (Smith 2004). The report, which runs to 1,000 pages and 109 recommendations is highly critical, not just of the old procedures for monitoring doctors' performance, but of the new procedures that were set to come into force in April 2005. Dame Smith did not believe that they would be adequate to protect the public from dysfunctional or under-performing doctors. In a letter to the Secretary of State for Health and to the Home Secretary (dated 29 November 2004), she described the GMC as focusing too strongly on the interests of doctors and not sufficiently on the protection of patients – in essence an organisation of doctors for doctors. At the same time, there is an imponderable question as to whether accountability and transparency can ever be made watertight enough to completely replace the need for some degree of trust (Smith 2005: 1). The correct balance has not yet been struck.

3 Home and away

Sharing care

Home at last

Susan tried very hard to resist the temptation, but she eventually gave way. Glad that Matthew wasn't around to see her do it, she went up to Daniel's room and checked the equipment over one more time. It was the third time that morning. The suction machine was working fine, as was the oxygen concentrator. The portable oxygen cylinders were stacked neatly in the corner of the room and Daniel's buggy had been adapted, so she could carry the cylinder easily on the tray underneath.

Daniel would be six months old in another week, and he had spent more than half of those months in the Albion. This afternoon he was finally coming home. This was going to be a very different homecoming from his first discharge from the Albion – this one had taken weeks of planning and was tinged with a new realism about what it was going to mean to care for a child with complex medical needs at home.

Over the past few months, Susan's world had been turned upside down. In the immediate aftermath of the nightmare consultation with Dr Hill, both Susan and Matthew had felt numb. That evening, looking at Daniel sucking hungrily on his bottle, Susan had alternated between disbelief that anything could really be wrong and overwhelming grief at the loss of the 'normal' child they had expected. She remembered her worst moment with absolute clarity. It was the morning after the diagnosis, and she had woken up and looked across at Daniel, sleeping peacefully in his cot, the bright autumn sunlight slanting in behind him, throwing shadows across his face. There were those few blissful seconds of sheer joy at the sight of him before the previous day's events had leapt back into her mind, and then the realisation had washed over her afresh, hitting her with sickening force in the pit of the stomach. The grief was even more overwhelming the second time than it had been the day before.

Having no idea who to turn to, she had phoned the respiratory ward at the Albion, desperately hoping that someone there would be able to say something to help ease the welling sense of panic. As luck would have it, Jackie Turner, the cystic fibrosis nurse specialist, was on the ward. She had ended up spending almost an hour on the phone to Jackie, and then Jackie had arranged for them to come and see Dr Sharpe, the consultant, at the end of the week.

Two weeks later, both Susan and Matthew had been on firmer ground. They'd seen Dr Sharpe, had several more conversations with Jackie, had a pile of leaflets and some books from the library and had spoken to another family with a child with cystic fibrosis. Their little girl was five years old and was doing really well. They also had an appointment booked for the following week to see Dr Khan, the consultant who was going to be looking after Daniel at St Michael's.

Susan's cousin, who had a farm in Suffolk, had suggested that she and Matthew really needed to get away for a few days with the children. He and his wife had a large sprawling house and there was always an endless stream of friends and family visiting from Ireland. Gratefully, they had taken him up on his offer, feeling much more confident because Daniel was thriving and gaining weight. It had seemed like just the slice of normality they needed. And then . . . disaster. Three days into their stay Daniel had developed a runny nose, cough and fever, and been admitted to the local hospital. And two days after that, they were back at the Albion.

The Albion – revisited

Susan knew they had been remarkably unlucky. Daniel had been infected with something called 'respiratory syncytial virus'. Apparently it was one of the commonest causes of wheezy episodes in babies and was not usually too troublesome. But it could result in much more severe problems, and in Daniel's case it had. He had gone on to get pneumonia, spent a period on a ventilator to help his breathing, and had been on oxygen ever since.

During the fourteen weeks that Daniel had spent at the Albion, Susan had become a different person. The Albion's Douglas Ward had, unavoidably, become a home from home, and she had become part of a new world and a new routine; one in which the day was punctuated not by when it was time to leave work, collect Sara from school and cook supper, but by the time of the next ward round, nursing handover and drug round. The daily currency of hospital life.

Through all this, Susan had developed a new language and a new set of parameters for a good day. She had a room in the building next door to the Albion, but spent only about six hours there, dead to the world every night. In the morning she'd rush back to the ward and check the number on the saturation monitor, the machine that recorded the oxygen levels in Daniel's blood. She'd ask the nurses about Daniel's 'overnight sats' (the monitor's figures that she'd missed while asleep), his breathing rate – all the tiny signs of recovery from his illness. And she'd gossip with the nurses, talk about what had happened in *EastEnders*, hear the latest about Sebastian's (he'd stopped being Dr Hill long ago) girlfriend. It wasn't normal life, but it was her new, alternative one.

It hadn't taken Susan long to discover that the Dr Hill who had told them Daniel's diagnosis was far from being the real Sebastian, whom she'd grown to like a lot. Underneath the brash exterior was an earnest young man who clung, against the odds, to naïve but strong ideals. And even though Susan wasn't much older than him, she'd felt strangely maternal when he was reproached on a ward round for not having the right set of results to hand and had blushed like a schoolgirl.

Matthew floated in and out of this hospital world like a reminder of a very distant one. Susan knew he was doing his best, rushing from work to get Sara from school, trying to maintain some kind of normality for her at home, ensuring that she had meals, homework done, her kit for gym. And while she and Daniel were in residence at the Albion, he would bring Sara down at the weekends and they would go to a museum or a café – something cheap – which made Susan feel an odd mix of better (for spending time with Sara), guilty (for how little time she had for her daughter) and sad (at leaving Daniel alone on the ward).

Susan dreamt of getting back to a better relationship with Matthew. She got so irritated when he didn't understand the nuances of the day-to-day changes in Daniel's condition, when he sat silently through meetings with staff at the Albion, looking at his son as if fearful that he might break, chewing his fingernails or fiddling with the car keys. His nervousness added to her feeling that she carried this burden alone.

She had talked to Jackie about the growing gulf between her and Matthew, even shared her fears that her second marriage was falling apart. And she confided in Jackie her mother's infuriating comment of the previous week: 'Isn't it unfair that now you've married one of our kind he's given your son this awful disease?' Susan could have told her mother, perhaps should have, for Matthew's sake, that the gene came from both of them. But she hadn't.

Jackie had been reassuring, suggested that all these things, even her mother's remark, were normal reactions to the stress of recent months. She'd said that things would settle down once Daniel was transferred from the Albion back to St Michael's, and they were not so far from home . . . and that was when Susan started to feel a new kind of panic.

Dr Khan

Mo Khan had just finished supper when Val Sharpe rang. Val and Mo had been registrars together at the Albion years earlier when both were pursuing careers in respiratory paediatrics. Mo was one of the brightest trainees on the circuit, had just completed a Ph.D. investigating the immune system in asthma, and word was that he was destined for a career as an academic clinician.

But soon after the birth of his third child, Mo had surprised everyone by deciding that teaching hospital paediatrics wasn't for him. It was the path of least resistance to keep taking the opportunities as they came – and they certainly came easily to him – but he'd made a conscious decision to call a halt and take stock. House prices in London were astronomical, and he was unimpressed with schools in the slightly run-down area where they had a small three-bedroom flat. He also worried about his elderly parents who lived in Brighton and were becoming increasingly frail.

Mo decided to move sideways: to do a year in general paediatrics and opt for a career as a paediatrician with a special interest in respiratory problems. He wanted to move out of London and to be closer to his parents. The St Michael's team were delighted when he applied for a consultant job there, his charisma, commitment and sound clinical judgement rapidly making him a lynchpin of the paediatric unit.

'Hi Val,' he grinned as he handed a tea towel to his wife and escaped the washing-up for the third night running. 'Long time no see. How's life at the centre of the paediatric universe these days?' The gentle tease had not been a good move. Ten minutes into the conversation, he'd been disabused of the notion that there were any fewer problems at the Albion than at St Michael's; they were simply different problems.

Eventually Val got to the point. Apologising for ringing him at home, she confessed that the call was work rather than social. Mo smiled wryly, never having been under any other illusion. First, would Mo come along to a workshop they were running on developing a children's health-care network across the region? They particularly wanted his input on how to smooth the path of children with cystic fibrosis. And second, on the subject of children with cystic fibrosis, there was one child in particular she'd been meaning to tell him about for several days.

'He had a pretty stormy course in the first few months,' Val explained, and ran quickly through his history. 'Anyway, the problem now is that we should be transferring him back to St Mike's, but the mother is point-blank refusing to move. She's got into this mindset that no one outside the Albion will be able to look after him. Says that St Mike's couldn't deal with him when he was born and had to tranfer him in here. Then the same thing happened when he was admitted to the local hospital near where they were staying in Suffolk . . . got bounced back to us within forty-eight hours. Of course, both those transfers were completely appropriate, but he's much better now, and they've got to make a relationship with you sooner or later.'

'Thanks Val,' Mo said. 'Always a pleasure to hear from you!'

'Oh sorry, Mo. There's one more thing. A good friend of hers died in St Mike's a couple of years ago. No idea of the details, but she obviously thinks the hospital was to blame somehow.'

'How far off discharge home is the child?' Mo asked.

'Well, he's pretty much ready, bar the fact that he'll need to go out on home oxygen, so that all needs to be set up,' Val replied.

'OK, well, if his mother is adamant about not coming into St Mike's at this stage, it will only make things worse if we push her. I know it's a bit unusual, but how about seeing if we can get him straight from the Albion to home? I'd need to talk to Penny. She's one of our community children's nurses. It's going to be a bit more complicated for her, and she'll obviously need to do the usual things – assessing the suitability of the house, organising home oxygen, and so on. But she's absolutely fantastic, and if anyone can build up the family's confidence in local services, she can. D'you think you'd be able to persuade the parents to at least attend a pre-discharge meeting at St Mike's with Penny, myself, the GP and so on? That way they'd be able to meet the key people, have a look round the ward and get a paediatric passport[1] so they can bypass A&E in an emergency.'

Val was sure that she could and thanked him profusely, feeling a great sense of relief as she put the phone down; she had moved her problem onto someone else's shoulders. Mo, for his part, decided that he'd paid a heavy price for escaping the washing-up again.

---

1 Most paediatric units issue cards – variously called 'green cards', 'paediatric passports' or 'emergency cards' – to children with chronic conditions such as severe asthma or cystic fibrosis.

Penny

Penny's own daughter was born on Boxing Day, with a rare cardiac condition that wasn't amenable to surgery. Christened Catherine, she survived just a week and was cremated in a small family service two days later. Penny hadn't started training as a nurse until she was twenty-six, three years after losing Catherine. Her husband had told her that this was a pathological response to losing their child, a substitute caring role, and that what she really needed was to have another baby. She told him that was nonsense and, in any event, he should look at his own response, which had been to hit the bottle – although in truth she thought that he'd have done that anyway. His father had also been an alcoholic. So, given the choice of giving up her career or her husband, she'd continued the former and given up on the latter. Twelve years later she hadn't regretted either decision, and was now married to a man nine years her senior, with three stepchildren from his previous marriage.

Penny's particular gift was an outgoing personality that made people at ease around her and an ability to charm the birds out of the trees, which was essential in her job. Only too often she would be left late on a Friday afternoon picking up the pieces when a child had been discharged precipitously from hospital without anyone being told – suddenly trying to magic a wheelchair or nasogastric feeding tube[1] or some other piece of essential equipment out of thin air before the weekend. However, she was getting the staff at St Mike's better trained, so this was a less frequent occurrence these days.

Dr Khan had briefed Penny about Daniel Johnson the morning after his call from Val Sharpe. Penny had managed to fit in a visit to see Susan at the Albion a couple of days later and, fortuitously, their shared Irish ancestry had given her an additional advantage in gaining Susan's trust. This had been important in the ensuing weeks as she had helped arrange Daniel's transfer home, taught Susan and Matthew all about how to manage home oxygen, liaised with Dr Khan and Dr Stebbing, the GP, to make sure Daniel's drugs were all organised and dealt with the plethora of other minutiae that were to make this discharge run smoothly.

---

1 Special tubes to feed straight into the stomach if a child cannot take food adequately by mouth.

A bit of a cough

Daniel had been home for ten weeks. Susan was surprised and relieved at just how smoothly things had gone, despite her worst fears. On the first afternoon, Penny had dropped in a couple of hours after they got him back and then popped in at gradually decreasing intervals as they found their feet. Susan had been to the GP practice to see Dr Stebbing – partly to top up Daniel's medicine supplies, but mostly to have a chat with him about Daniel's eczema. Having cystic fibrosis didn't stop him from having other common baby ailments as well. She had also had a couple of visits from the health visitor, who had helped her iron out some problems with Daniel's feeding, and he was now gaining weight really well. The best day had been when they'd gone for a routine follow-up appointment with Dr Khan, when Daniel had been home for eight weeks. He had been really impressed with how they were all doing and even thought that it might not be too long before Daniel could come off home oxygen.

The first hint of trouble came one Friday afternoon, when Daniel started coughing again and developed a low-grade fever. Other than that, he seemed quite cheerful and had demolished his lunch with gusto. Penny was away for a long weekend, so Susan decided to ring the practice and talk to Dr Stebbing.

Jack Stebbing's surgery was already running late when Katie, his receptionist buzzed through to tell him that Mrs Johnson was coming in with her little boy who had cystic fibrosis, and she hoped that was alright.

'Yes, of course,' Jack said. 'But would you mind calling Liz for me and telling her I'm running late and I don't think I'll be home in time to pick David up from Judo?' Cowardice being the better part of valour, he decided against making the call himself, since this was the third time this week he'd failed on a home commitment. Hardly an unprecedented event, but there were limits to even Liz's patience, and he knew that Katie would not get the earful that he would.

When Susan arrived, Jack still had two people to see. He spent almost half an hour with a woman who had a four-month-old son and who clearly had terrible post-natal depression. Her son wasn't ill, but she was, and he couldn't have cut their consultation any shorter. He felt fairly confident about prescribing Prozac for her, knowing it was quite safe even for mothers who were breast-feeding. However, the more problematic issue was that she clearly needed to be seen in the Mother and Baby Rapid Assessment Unit where they specialised in managing post-natal depression. He had to get a referral faxed through as quickly as possible, and it was Sod's Law that she'd appeared in an overbooked Friday-afternoon surgery, when the chances of him catching someone before the weekend were diminishing by the minute.

Immediately before calling Susan in, he'd seen Mr Powell, an elderly man whose wife had Parkinson's disease. Mr Powell had read over the weekend about stem-cell treatment and a new drug that the government was deciding whether to make available. He'd said he'd pay for either of these if they could help his wife get better and asked Dr Stebbing what 'NICE' was.

Again, there was too much to sort out in one go. Dr Stebbing knew it was too long since he'd seen Mrs Powell and he ought to organise a home visit. He knew that she'd be long gone before stem-cell treatment became a reality and suspected she was already too disabled for the new drug to be any good to her even if NICE – the National Institute for Clinical Excellence[1] – eventually recommended its use, which he doubted they would.

He felt a mix of irritation that, again, media hype promised cures to desperate patients when the treatment had been tested on three Californian mice, and irritation at himself for having been caught off guard yet again by a clued-up carer. He did as well as anyone could about keeping up to date, through the mandatory continuing professional development programme. But still it was impossible to stay one step ahead on every new treatment that hit the medical and, worse still, the national press.

'Mrs Johnson, do come in,' he said, as he ushered Susan into the room. He knew from the pre-discharge meeting at St Mike's that Susan was liable to be pretty edgy and, although she'd been to see him about various minor issues, this was the first really significant consultation since Daniel's discharge. It was important that it went well.

'I gather that Daniel's a bit off colour.' Rapidly appraising Daniel as he sat in his buggy he thought that, apart from the tell-tale nasal cannula[2] and oxygen cylinder, Daniel was looking remarkably well.

'Well, he's been doing fine, and I feel a bit silly bringing him in now. It's just that he's developed a bit of a cough, and his temperature was up earlier on. He seems to have settled a bit now.'

'No, no, not at all,' Jack said. 'You did absolutely the right thing to bring him.'

He examined Daniel carefully. Apart from the slight temperature, there was nothing else to find. His breathing was normal, his chest was quite clear, and there were no signs of infection anywhere else.

1 See Chapter 5
2 Tubing that delivers oxygen from the cylinder to the baby's nose.

'Given his history, we'd better give him some antibiotics just to be on the safe side,' Jack said, writing a prescription. 'The pharmacy down the street is open late, so you should be able to pick them up there.'

'Thank you, Dr Stebbing,' Susan said, clearly relieved.

'And don't worry,' Jack added. 'I'm doing the Saturday-morning emergency surgery tomorrow, so if you're at all worried just bring him back in.'

A turn for the worse

That night, Daniel's breathing rate shot up, and he was feverish and sweaty. Susan saw the skin between his ribs draw in oddly with the effort of each breath and knew from experience that this was a bad sign. Yet she still hoped they might be able to cope at home.

She decided to call the surgery and talk to Dr Stebbing. But the practice had a new night service where you left your number and a doctor phoned back. After an interminable period that was actually only three to four minutes, someone called back and started to ask about Daniel. What was his date of birth? Had he ever been in hospital before? Was he on any medicine? Had he ever suffered from cough or shortage of breath previously?

'Look, this is hopeless. Never mind, we'll sort it out ourselves,' Susan said, and slammed the phone down.

'Matt, we have to get him back to the Albion,' she said. 'I'll get him ready while you take Sara next door.'

'No Susan,' Matthew said. 'We should take him to St Mike's.'

'Look Matt, they won't be able to deal with this. I need to get him to somewhere I can trust. Don't make this more difficult for me. Please, just hurry up with Sara.'

Matthew didn't move. 'Susan this isn't about you. It's about Daniel. And it's about me as well. Daniel is my son too.'

'Yes, but you . . . but, I mean I . . . well, it's me who's been looking after him . . .'

'What you've been doing is shutting me out . . . carrying on as if I don't exist or have any feelings in this. So why don't you take Sara next door, while I get Daniel ready, and then we'll go to St Mike's.'

St Michael's

When they got to Rainbow Ward, the children's ward at St Michael's, Susan was surprised to discover they were expecting them. Matthew had apparently phoned ahead whilst she was taking Sara next door.

A rather young-looking nurse, who introduced herself as Mandy Watson, showed them to a cot and started to check Daniel's observations: his temperature, pulse and breathing rate. Susan thought she was too young to be qualified – that she was probably a student – and hoped that someone more senior would arrive soon.

'Have you been training long?' she asked, nonetheless quite impressed with the calm and confident way in which Mandy was rapidly switching Daniel from his own cylinder oxygen to wall oxygen, attaching an oximeter (the device to monitor his blood oxygen levels) and gently positioning him so that he seemed a little more comfortable almost immediately.

'Actually I'm the senior staff nurse here,' Mandy smiled as she pulled down the top of the plastic apron she was wearing to reveal her name badge. 'Big disadvantage being a baby face! Not good for the gravitas, but can't quite swing half-price tickets in the cinema.'

Susan flushed with embarrassment, just as the paediatric registrar arrived and had a quick conversation with Mandy. Susan had been rehearsing in her mind the best way to ask to be transferred back to the Albion where they had all Daniel's records and would know how to deal with this. She had to find some way of asking without offending this new set of strangers. But before she got a chance to frame the question the registrar explained that she had already heard about the day's events over the phone from Matthew and had also got quite a lot of information from Daniel's notes. She was just going to listen to his chest, and it would probably be sensible to pop a drip up, give him some medicine via a face mask and order an X-ray. Then she would go through everything with them in a bit more detail.

Susan realised that things were now out of her hands. Turning to Matthew she said, 'I'm sorry, Matt . . . about . . . well everything. He's going to be alright here, isn't he?'

'Yes love,' Matthew replied. 'We're all going to be alright.'

Cut! Rewind

Susan and Matthew had moved on an inexorable path from sharing the joy of their first child together to a world that neither of them had ever imagined. As their expectations of life as a normal family were gradually torn away from them, they clung on to any alternative reality that was able to provide them with some security on their precipitous journey. For Susan, the Albion had become a critical part of that alternative reality and to let go of it was both frightening and painful.

This chapter highlights several important issues. A central theme, as in Chapter 2, is the importance of communication; but this time the communication is between organisations as well as individuals. Alongside communication, a new theme emerges: the importance of trust. Discussion about this will be opened here, but revisited throughout the book because, like communication, it is one of the bedrocks on which health care must stand.

In this scenario, we illustrated how good communication between primary, secondary and tertiary care was able to make Daniel's transition run more smoothly. When we played this particular episode out on stage at GOSH, we ran the story differently and illustrated the converse. How poor communication between health-care professionals resulted in increased distress for the Johnsons and destroyed their trust in St Michael's. In the same way that some of the process problems outlined in the first chapter were a contributory factor to the failure of communication between Sebastian and the Johnsons, so too poor communication between primary, secondary and tertiary health-care settings can result in failures of trust.

Fragmentation and poor communication, whether between primary, secondary and tertiary health-care services, or between health, social services and education can cause more than a breakdown in trust. Such failures contribute to the broader problems of caring for children with complex needs at home, and supporting their families. Good communication between services is also a crucial prerequisite in protecting vulnerable children from harm, and we will discuss the catastrophic consequences when this goes wrong, and some of the measures being taken to develop better integrated care systems.

As a backdrop to all these issues, there are the broader societal questions of how we value children, how we care for individuals with complex health needs and, at the end of the day, how medical advances push us to make increasingly difficult life and death decisions.

THE HEALTH-CARE SYSTEM: CARE IN THE COMMUNITY

When Susan and Matthew took Daniel home from the Albion for the first time, they hoped and believed that they were taking home a normal baby. They had every reason to expect that life was going to get back on track, just as they had planned it in the months and years that they prayed for Susan to conceive. The second time they left the Albion, it was with a baby who was 'technology-dependent', a term used to describe an increasing number of children who need 'both a medical device to compensate for the loss of a vital body function, and ongoing nursing care.' They were going to need support from a huge range of professionals – many of whom were based in the community rather than the hospital.

Medical advances in the care of premature and seriously ill children have led to an increasing number of such children; a study in 2000 estimated that there were approximately 6,000 technology dependent children across the United Kingdom, and numbers have almost inevitably risen since then. The cost of looking after these children at home may be as high as 150,000 pounds per child per annum (Glendinning et al. 2001). Research highlights some worrying and contentious issues (Wang and Barnard 2004, Kirk and Glendinning 2004). Most importantly, it suggests that development of appropriate community-based services is variable around the country and, in some areas, has not kept pace with the needs of this group.

In this chapter, we will discuss some of the research and policy that is relevant to the care of children with complex health needs at home. But it is always valuable to ground theory in reality, and we have been fortunate in having help and insights from one particular couple whose daughter, Katie, had a rare and complex medical condition. Sadly, Katie died when she was just under two years old, but her parents, Tracey and Keith McBride, hope that by sharing their experience with readers of this book, they may be able to make a small difference to other children and to their families and carers.

Although some of the problems outlined below are specific to children with complex medical needs, many will also be familiar to other families and carers; first to families looking after children with severe physical or learning disabilities, and second to those looking after parents or partners who are disabled, technology dependent or dependent on other forms of care.

Problems in the provision of care at home

So what are the key issues for families and carers and for the professionals involved in supporting them at home?

Whose choice?

> I think the thing that I feel . . . people think that you're a parent,
> you're just here to care for your child whatever happens . . . I felt
> I was the person coordinating all the care and it was a mega-
> weight when you're under stress . . . it gets a heavy load to carry.
> (Kirk and Glendinning 2004: 213)

Parents want to have their children at home, and rightly so. We know
that home is the best place for a child to be, and both health and social
policy has been directed at shortening the length of time that children
spend in hospitals. But are our health and social services adequately
resourced and organised to support parents in caring for these children
at home? And is it right to expect parents to just take on the burden
of this care, regardless of the emotional, financial and social cost to
them and their other children?

The practical reality is that whilst health-care professionals choose
to take on a clinical role, parents of sick or disabled children are not
given this choice. Many families in the studies referenced above felt
there was no negotiation, merely an expectation, that they would take
on a variety of technical and clinical tasks – sometimes painful and
distressing ones – alongside parenting and advocating for their child
and coordinating the input of the multitude of other people involved
in their care.

> I remember thinking how could the local hospital send us home
> knowing I would have to pass nasogastric tubes on my daugh-
> ter,[1] sometimes on my own, while my husband was at work?
> 'You could come to ambulatory care and we could put it back
> for you,' the staff nurse said. The thought of driving twelve
> miles anytime of day and night – perhaps numerous times –
> was unthinkable . . . but we couldn't afford for our daughter to
> have her continual milk feed disrupted, because she would have
> no chance of gaining weight. That's when I realised there was no

1 The feeding tube which needs to go through the nose into the stomach of a
child who can't take food by mouth.

continued

immediate cure and that we would be coping – or at least trying to cope – with her illness at home.

Medical supplies were, on the whole, provided on a rolling stock every few weeks, but trying to make slight alterations was often met with difficulty. So too was the process of reordering drugs from the local pharmacy, only to find out that the alterations in dosage made during the last hospital admission had not been communicated to the GP practice and then the pharmacy.

At home, the sweet child's bedroom we had decorated suddenly started to look clinical – and like a medical store room.

(Tracey McBride, mother of a child
with complex health needs)

Impact on the family

Notwithstanding the willingness of most parents to shoulder the burden of care for their children, it is easy to underestimate the impact of the unremitting round-the-clock demands. Both parents and professionals describe difficulties in accessing respite and support services as one of the biggest problems. Parents may go for months without ever getting a full night's sleep, being woken by alarms on machines, and often just not being able to experience normal deep sleep because of the need for constant vigilance. There is frequently social isolation, because it is hard or even impossible to go out with the child and equally difficult to find people who are able to babysit without recourse to specially recruited and trained support workers. Holidays, if possible at all, have to be organised around accessibility to a nearby hospital.

The potential impact on parents, on siblings, and on family relationships is self-evident. It is easy for carers to become exhausted, burnt out and depressed.

Mind the gap

Despite the aspiration to produce seamless services, fragmentation of care is an ongoing nightmare for families. Disputes between acute and community trusts, GPs, health authorities and social services create major stress, whether in relation to supplies of equipment and consumables or provision of short-term care and support.

There is also often lack of clarity about who has duty of care, who is leading on specific aspects and who the family should call in a crisis. At one extreme, parents can be overloaded with visits from professionals, with no coordination of care and, at the other, can have no one to turn to when they need help. Communication between the hospital and community professionals is frequently poor, with community teams not always being informed about readmissions, discharges or new treatment regimes.

The paediatric nurse who looked after our daughter Katie was very sympathetic and gave emotional support, but due to the rarity of Katie's illness we often felt alone as parents.

So many of the problems we faced left us feeling ALONE, a word I used numerous times. A word I used to all the multidisciplinary persons involved in Katie's care, a word I used when crying on the phone to our local hospital and the main children's hospital. As we were intelligent, practical, caring and willing parents, I believe we were often left to be doctor, nurse, secretary, coordinator and then parents whilst being ALONE.

(Tracey and Keith McBride, parents of a child with complex health needs)

The theme that recurs in every study, every document and every policy about supporting patients and families is the need for a key worker, someone the family knows and trusts, who can find out the answers to questions, even if they don't have the information themselves. In some instances, the role also blurs into one of advocacy for the family, but one could argue that these could, and perhaps should, be separate roles. An advocate key worker, who may be a parent themselves, can be impartial and, in some respects, can share the experience with the family and can be a representative for them, providing family support, counselling and resource advice. The case coordinator is someone who is probably a professional and can be the single point of contact for the family and steer them through the maze of care. The quotes above highlight the fact that both roles are essential.

Without doubt, where there is a good community children's nursing team, problems are reduced. People like Penny are in the best position to help organise ordering of supplies and to provide a link between hospital and community services. Unfortunately, this is not the whole answer. First, there is a national shortage of community children's nurses (CCNs) and, hence, a postcode lottery as to whether there is a local service available at all. Second, the CCNs may be based in either the acute trust or in the community. There can be pluses and minuses for each. For example, if they are based in the acute trust, they may have better links with the paediatricians and inpatient services, are more likely to be well informed about admissions and to be able to help with discharges. On the other hand, they may not be as well able to push for services and supplies that are normally funded by the community budget. A fuller explanation of these 'divided camps' and the plans for improving the situation are outlined below.

The plight of the GP

A crucially important player in Daniel's care at home is, of course, Jack Stebbing, his GP. GPs see large numbers of people and are expected to know how to deal with them all. But how can they keep a broad enough knowledge base to cope with everyone, from the very young to the very old, from those with sore throats, to children like Daniel and to those with cancer? And, in the midst of this, how can they also find time to give health-promotion advice, sort out whether people need Prozac or psychological support, arrange for this (often through serious obstacles and long waits) and give evidence to the committees that decide whether people like Mrs Powell are eligible for new drugs for Parkinson's? And this is not to mention having enough spare time to input to their local Primary Care Trust, manage their budgets and respond to soaring numbers of appraisals and evaluations? No wonder Jack struggled to keep on top of the information load and to stay abreast of new advances in a huge diversity of fields.

The pressures on GPs are undeniable. A Royal College of General Practitioners report in 2002 (Stress and General Practice) concluded that stress was endemic in general practice. The data was alarming. A survey of GP retirement found that a quarter planned to retire before the age of sixty with 'health, including stress' contributing to 36 per cent of these decisions. A further study found that half of GPs had been categorised as suffering from probable borderline or more severe anxiety, and a quarter as suffering from at least borderline depression. In other words, those with front-line responsibility for looking after the health of the nation are themselves about twice as likely as the general population to be at risk of psychiatric illness and to retire early as a result.

So who is looking after them? Often no one but themselves, with GPs tending to self-medicate, women more so than men. Indeed female GPs reported higher stress levels, with fear of being assaulted on night calls and conflict between work–home lives being a major source of anxiety. The suicide of Dawn Harris in 2003 was attributed to depression due to the stress of her job and the tension of being a perfectionist who felt unable to do enough for her patients.

Dawn Harris's death came in the wake of reports that British GPs spend an average of only nine minutes with each patient and fears that it will be a long time before any new investment eases their burdens and frees them up to see patients for longer. Many find the extra bureaucracy of the new systems arduous and do not see changes happening fast enough. Meanwhile, a recruitment crisis in primary care looms as the large group of Asian doctors who came to the UK in the 1960s, and make up a quarter of all GPs in some areas, retire. Alongside all this, GPs are expected to offer appointments within forty-eight hours or lose points in performance ratings. Tension is understandable.

Improving the provision of care, and not just at home

When it comes to capturing media and public interest, hospital care has always held centre stage. Debates about the government's success in improving health care have tended to focus most strongly on progress in reducing trolley waits in A&E and waiting lists for operations. The documentaries that attract the highest viewer ratings are those that showcase miraculous operations and cutting-edge treatments. Yet hospital care represents only the tip of the iceberg of the health needs of the nation. Eighty-two per cent of contacts between patients and the NHS take place outside hospital – with GPs, practice nurses, community nurses, community dentists and a host of others (Department of Health 2004).

This means that to improve the care of children like Daniel, there have to be fundamental changes in the way in which health care is organised. These changes are underway. First, there have been major changes in the way in which health-care services are planned and commissioned. Second, there have been some much more specific changes, focused on the particular needs of children and young people.

Shifting the balance of power

As the NHS passed its first half century, successive governments had faced an increasing challenge in providing a health-care service that would meet the more rapidly changing demands of current society. Having published the NHS Plan (NHS Executive 2000), the Labour Government had left itself with the dilemma of meeting a large number of targets in a relatively short time frame. The United Kingdom was not alone in its struggle with these issues. In Canada, a health-care evaluation at much the same time identified a rather similar cocktail of problems: long waiting lists, overspending, a focus on access at cost of quality, staff shortages and low morale (Dixon 2001).

Recognising the problems of driving change through a strongly centrally managed bureaucracy, one of the major planks of the Government's plan was to try to decentralise power through a new structure. In 2001, it published *Shifting the Balance of Power* (Department of Health 2001b). The aim of this reorganisation was to bring together GPs and community health services into newly formed Primary Care Trusts (PCTs). These PCTs would then have responsibility for assessing the needs of their local population and ensuring delivery of all necessary services, either by providing them directly or by commissioning them from local hospital trusts. Meanwhile the ninety-six Health Authorities, which had previously managed many of these functions, were replaced by twenty-eight Strategic Health Authorities (SHAs). Instead of money being channelled through the Health Authorities to the acute hospitals, 75 per cent of it was devolved straight to the PCTs. The SHAs stepped back into a different role, managing the performance of the newly formed PCTs and NHS Trusts (see Figure 3.1).

In many sectors, there was dismay at the prospect of yet another reorganisation (Smith, Walshe and Hunter 2001). Policy-makers, GPs and managers all worried about the 'change fatigue' within the Health Service, the ability of the newly formed PCTs to take on this challenge and the fact that they were going to be poachers and gamekeepers – both providing and commissioning services. The task set for the PCTs was certainly ambitious. As relatively new organisations, they had to hit the ground running in meeting the local health-care requirements, in many cases without having the necessary management structures in place to tackle this huge agenda.

So was this new system able to help Daniel, his family and the many other chronically ill patients and families trying to access health-care services at home? In theory, the new system should have given Jack

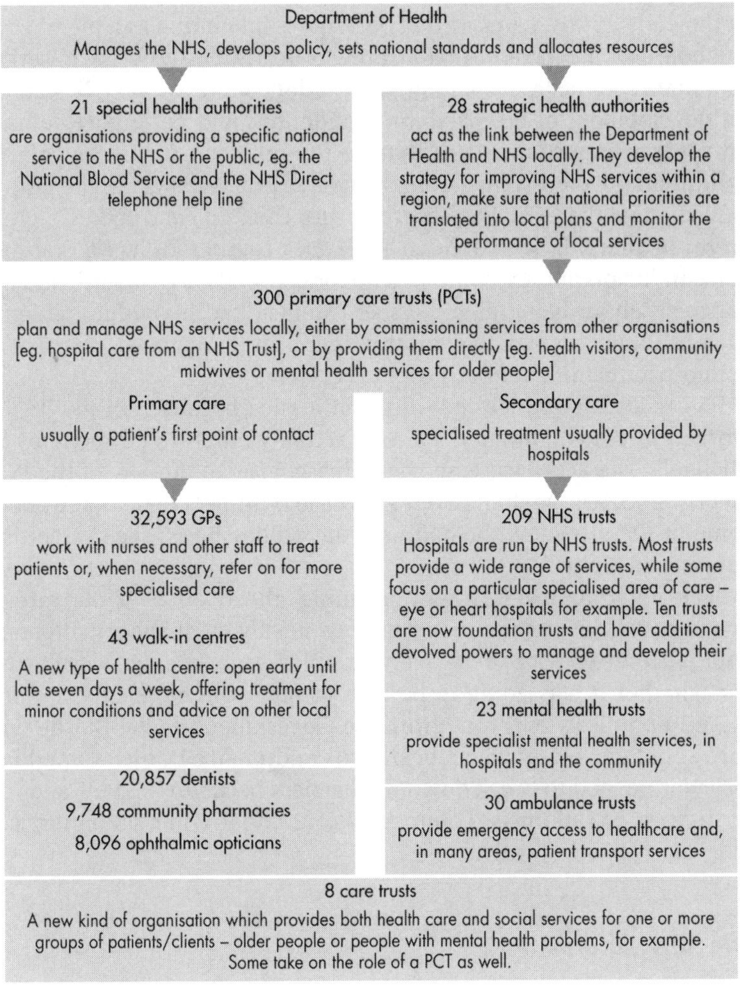

Department of Health
Manages the NHS, develops policy, sets national standards and allocates resources

21 special health authorities
are organisations providing a specific national service to the NHS or the public, eg. the National Blood Service and the NHS Direct telephone help line

28 strategic health authorities
act as the link between the Department of Health and NHS locally. They develop the strategy for improving NHS services within a region, make sure that national priorities are translated into local plans and monitor the performance of local services

300 primary care trusts (PCTs)
plan and manage NHS services locally, either by commissioning services from other organisations [eg. hospital care from an NHS Trust], or by providing them directly [eg. health visitors, community midwives or mental health services for older people]

Primary care
usually a patient's first point of contact

Secondary care
specialised treatment usually provided by hospitals

32,593 GPs
work with nurses and other staff to treat patients or, when necessary, refer on for more specialised care

43 walk-in centres
A new type of health centre: open early until late seven days a week, offering treatment for minor conditions and advice on other local services

20,857 dentists
9,748 community pharmacies
8,096 ophthalmic opticians

209 NHS trusts
Hospitals are run by NHS trusts. Most trusts provide a wide range of services, while some focus on a particular specialised area of care – eye or heart hospitals for example. Ten trusts are now foundation trusts and have additional devolved powers to manage and develop their services

23 mental health trusts
provide specialist mental health services, in hospitals and the community

30 ambulance trusts
provide emergency access to healthcare and, in many areas, patient transport services

8 care trusts
A new kind of organisation which provides both health care and social services for one or more groups of patients/clients – older people or people with mental health problems, for example. Some take on the role of a PCT as well.

Figure 3.1 The NHS in England.

Source: *State of Healthcare* report, 2004. Reproduced with kind permission of the Healthcare Commission.

Stebbing, Penny and the other people directly involved in looking after Daniel more influence in pushing for resources for him with the PCT. In practice, no single solution is a 'cure-all' for complex problems, and the front-line limitations can best be illustrated by a momentary 'revisit' to our fictional players.

Jack's practice had been one of the early fund-holding practices back in the early 1990s. Later he had been quite influential as a member of the board of his local Primary Care Group (PCG) – the organisation that preceded the PCT. He thought he'd done quite a good job, leading on development of the paediatric guidelines and getting agreement on several important issues that he thought had made the care of children more consistent across the twelve practices within the group. However, as the PCG was absorbed into the PCT, and the PCT grew larger by merging with another PCT, Jack found that he had far less voice in the organisation. He was no longer on the PCT board, and his concerns about being able to meet the needs of individual patients such as Daniel seemed to get lost in much larger agendas, such as the commissioning of complex hospital services.

Penny also found she had little influence because, although she worked in the community, she was actually employed directly by St Michael's, the acute trust, so she didn't get invited to any of the PCT meetings. Often she didn't even know the right people to talk to about some of the problems she had on a day-to-day basis, such as getting equipment funded.

Jack felt that his PCT was storming ahead on a whole raft of agendas, and he was impressed at how quickly the management team had got to grips with some really complex problems. He wasn't sure yet whether it was going to be able to meet the huge expectations placed upon it by everyone from the Government down. But he was sure about one thing: when it came to children like Daniel, something else was needed to break down the barriers between the PCT and the acute trust, to rationalise communications and to commission services in a more joined-up way.

The new GP contract

The new GP contract represents one of the most fundamental changes in primary care since the launch of the NHS in 1948. For the first time, money will follow patients rather than GPs, with the new contract being between the PCT and the practice, rather than with individual GPs. This rationale for this change is to generate services that can be delivered more flexibly through a team-based approach, using whichever staff and skill mix is most appropriate. If a GP leaves, they could be replaced by a salaried partner, additional practice nurses, community pharmacists or any other staff member.

GPs stand to gain financially, but to do so will need to offer a broader range of services. They can choose to deliver three different levels of care, from basic 'bread and butter' services, through additional services (for example, childhood vaccinations and cervical screening), to enhanced services such as minor surgery. There is also scope for GPs to develop special interests in particular fields, such as gynaecology, diabetes, skin problems, and to deliver services within the practice so that fewer patients have to attend hospital Outpatients. In effect, GPs will be rewarded for providing quality services that best meet the needs of their patient population.

Needless to say, there are many complexities and potential pitfalls. First, the need to measure quality and adherence to targets is implicit in the plan. Since the proposal spells out seventy-six quality indicators in ten clinical domains of care, fifty-six in organisational areas, four assessing patients' experience and a number of indicators for additional services, this task will not be straightforward (Shekelle 2003). And then there is always the question of what happens to the non-targeted aspects of practice that are not linked to financial reward; might these suffer as a result of an understandable emphasis on the identified targets?

But, perhaps most controversially, GPs under the new contract can opt out of providing out-of-hours cover for a penalty of 6,000 pounds, leaving the PCT to provide emergency cover and any additional services that GPs decide not to undertake. This could lead to greater fragmentation of these aspects of care and to more people like the Johnsons making out-of-hours calls to contracted night services with no access to their medical records. And this is clearly not the path to improving patient trust.

Managed clinical networks

Linked groups of health professionals and organisations from primary, secondary and tertiary care working in a co-ordinated manner, unconstrained by existing professional and [organisational] boundaries to ensure equitable provision of high quality, clinically effective services.
(Definition of 'Managed clinical networks',
The Scottish Office 1998)

Back at St Michael's, Mo Khan had been a bit dubious about getting drawn into Val Sharpe's workshop about forming a children's network. He'd been to too many meetings recently about joined-up working and smoothing the patient journey. It all felt rather vague, and he couldn't quite square the vision with day-to-day life at St Michael's, the usual problems of shortages of nurses, inexperienced junior doctors who were now all working shorter hours and a cramped Outpatient Department that needed to be redesigned to be more child-friendly. But in the end, Mo decided to go, because he was convinced that some kind of change was needed, and maybe this time it was really going to happen.

In almost every sphere of life, we are part of informal networks. We all have friends and colleagues that we phone for advice and bounce ideas off and who we can draft in to help with particular problems. Whether it's a case of phoning another parent in the National Childbirth Trust (NCT) group who's had a baby with bad colic, e-mailing a fellow architect who's had to deal with a similar bridge-building project or borrowing a mechanic from your cousin's garage because your own is off sick, these connections are crucial to all our lives. What are the unifying features of these links? First, they are informal and spontaneous; second, they are not hierarchical but are instead reciprocal relationships; third, they are not dependent on organisational management or financial arrangements; and, fourth, they are not competitive. And finally, of course, they work!

Is it possible to set up more formal networks that have all the advantages of an informal network, but with a clearer framework? There are benefits in making a network more formal, outcomes that could not be achieved through the informal relationships described above. For example, by having some rules and shared standards, similar high-calibre clinical guidelines can be delivered on every site within the network, from primary through to tertiary care. The first example of this was through cancer networks, and other network models have flowed from some of this early learning. Joint training can take place, pathways of care can be defined and particular types of activity can take place on different sites. For example, specialist services can be delivered much closer to home in the local hospital rather than only at the tertiary centre.

In order to achieve this, member organisations need to surrender sovereignty to achieve shared objectives (NHS Confederation 2001b), and the cultural change that this implies is one of the real challenges in making this model successful. Another huge challenge is in deciding how 'managed' the network should be. For example, where operation of services is separated from ownership and operation of the infra-structure, there is potential for organisational mayhem, as has been the case with privatisation of the railways, where different services need to connect with each other, share ticketing arrangements, and so on (NHS Confederation 2001b). Thus, there needs to be an optimum level of hierarchical control and accountability, without losing the flexibility and fluidity of the network concept.

The concept of paediatric networks has been well established in North America for some time. For example, the Children's Hospital of Philadelphia operates through a number of networked hospitals closer to children's homes. Recently this model has been adopted in London, with the Children's and Young People's Partnership for Health, linking GOSH and some of its neighbouring district general and PCT partners in a newly formed network. Whilst the London model is of a more formally managed structure, Partners in Paediatrics (PiP) is a much larger, but more diffuse model linking nineteen trusts including Birmingham, Manchester and Liverpool.

An early lesson from PiP, and one echoed in the NHS Confederation's discussion document about clinical networks, is that the current mechanisms for commissioning services still do not fit well with a network concept, because they purchase services individually rather than on a networked basis (Spencer and Cropper 2004). So, if networks are a step in the right direction, what else is needed to provide truly 'joined-up' services? This is an important question for all health-care services, but particularly so for children's services, where failures of communication within and between statutory services can lead to tragic results.

Children's trusts

> Victoria, she was my blood, my own child. But I'm thinking about other people's children. We all have the same blood. We have to protect our children and stop this happening.
> (Berthe Climbié, mother of Victoria, *BBC News*, September 2001)

Victoria Climbié was born in November 1991 in the Ivory Coast, and died in February 2000 in St Mary's Hospital in London after suffering months of neglect and torture. She was eight years old, and her parents had sent her to England for a better life. The perpetrators of this appalling abuse were her great-aunt Marie-Therese Kouao, and Kouao's boyfriend Carl Manning.

What is the connection between Daniel's story and Victoria's – one a fictional story of a child with a chronic illness, the other an all too real story of a previously healthy child whose death represented a failure of multiple individuals and systems? Whilst for Daniel and Victoria the stakes were very different, both needed good communication to take place not just within the Health Service, but between Health and Social Services. Both needed appropriately resourced children's services, which were not constrained by organisational boundaries or divisive commissioning systems. And both needed inter-agency collaboration to ensure that staff were trained and performing to an appropriate standard.

> Victoria was known to no fewer than four social services departments, three housing departments, two specialist child protection teams of the metropolitan Police. Furthermore, she was admitted to two different hospitals because of concerns that she was being deliberately harmed and was referred to a specialist Children and families centre managed by the NSPCC. All of this between 26th April 1999 and 25th February 2000.
>
> What transpired during this period can only be described as a catalogue of administrative, managerial and professional failure by the services charged with her safety.
>
> In Brent, Victoria's case was given no fewer than 5 "unique" reference numbers. Retrieving files, I was told, was like the national lottery, and with similar odds.
>
> (Lord Laming 2003)

In January 2003, Lord Laming, who had headed up the public inquiry into Victoria's death, made a series of recommendations for radical changes to the delivery of children's welfare services. His report was followed in autumn 2003 by a Green Paper *Every Child Matters* (Department for Education and Skills and Department of Health 2003) and then The Children Bill in March 2004, both aimed at improving opportunities for children and protecting them from risk. For example, the Bill sets out plans for electronic files on every child in the country, to identify and keep track of those at risk from abuse, neglect, school exclusion, offending and social exclusion.

One planned outcome is the development of children's trusts. The main purpose of these trusts, which will be run by local government, will be to secure integrated commissioning of services across all the statutory agencies, including Health, Education and Social Services. It is planned that they will also provide common assessment frameworks, information-sharing systems and joint training. Individual organisations within this larger commissioning group can still be separately managed, but with the pooling of the budget and of information, it is hoped that thinking will be joined up and that children won't fall through the cracks.

If children's trusts are able to deliver on Alan Milburn's statement that, 'in future services must be centred not around any particular organisation but around the interests of the child' (Milburn 2003), then the interests of Daniel and of other 'at risk' children like Victoria will be well served. This is true regardless of whether the need is for provision of respite care for families of sick children, or well-trained and proactive social workers who might spot the signs of abuse before another tragedy occurs.

Box 3.1 Learning points for everyone: protecting children

- Protecting children is everyone's business, whether you are a health-care professional, work in another agency or are a member of the public.
- Anyone who works in a childcare setting has a responsibility to stay up to date in child-protection training. You should be familiar with the local policies and procedures for dealing with any situation in which child abuse is suspected.
- For professional staff: ensure you have read 'What to Do if You're Worried a Child is Being Abused' on the Department of Health web site: <http://www.dh.gov.uk>.
- For members of the public: read 'Are You Worried about a Child?' on the NSPCC web site: <http://www.nspcc.org.uk>, or ring the twenty-four-hour child-protection helpline on 0808 800 5000. If in doubt – act, don't wait. Advice is confidential, but your actions could save a child's life.

THE SOCIETAL CONTEXT: THE CHILD FIRST AND ALWAYS?

Valuing children

'The Child First and Always' is the motto of Great Ormond Street Hospital, and remains as valid a guiding principle today as it has been throughout the history of the hospital.

All parents will recognise that nothing and no one is more important to them than their children. In December 2003, Paul Randall, a forty-nine-year old man from Kent, put his kidney up for auction on e-bay. Mr Randall's daughter, aged six at that time, has cerebral palsy, and he was prepared to risk prosecution and his own health, in order to pay for therapy that he believed would help her walk. There are legion stories of parents making the most extraordinary sacrifices and, in extreme cases, laying down their lives for the sake of their children. The survival of the species – indeed of every species – is dependent on the ferocity with which bears will defend their cubs and mothers their children. This is a basic biological instinct.

Society is not driven by biological instinct, but by financial, political and cultural expedience, so it is perhaps not surprising that children have not always held the same central position in society that they hold in the hearts of their parents. In July 2000, the *British Medical Journal* (*BMJ*) published a paper written by ten of the most prominent leaders in children's health care (Aynsley-Green et al. 2000). Professor Al Aynsley-Green, the first author, was then Director of Research and Development at GOSH. The paper criticised the Government for failing to give children's health care high enough priority on its policy agenda.

Exactly one year later, in July 2001, Ian Kennedy's report into children's heart surgery at Bristol Royal Infirmary was published (see Chapter 1). The report – *Learning from Bristol* (Bristol Royal Infirmary 2001) – found that over thirty children had died unnecessarily as a result of system failures, inadequate paediatric provision and a 'club culture' that generated an imbalance of power and poor teamwork. Some of these issues, which will be discussed in more detail in Chapter 7, have had far-reaching consequences, not only for children's services, but also for the entire practice of medicine. However, a powerful message from the report was that children's health-care services were fragmented and uncoordinated, and that they had to be given higher priority in the NHS – a striking echo of the earlier *BMJ* paper. In response to the report, the Health Secretary announced the immediate appointment of Professor Al Aynsley-Green as National Clinical Director for Children's Health-Care Services.

In September 2002, Professor Aynsley-Green gave a public lecture at GOSH entitled 'The Child First and Always: Is It?' (Aynsley-Green 2002). Much of the content of this lecture has subsequently been reproduced in an article in *Current Paediatrics* (Aynsley-Green 2004). The lecture provided a historical overview that catalogued a bleak and sobering account of childhood through the ages, frequently marked by brutality and exploitation. It was not until around 1800, when Jean-Jacques Rousseau argued specifically for the rights of the child, that a more enlightened view started to emerge. Nonetheless, through the Victorian era, as industrialisation and urbanisation were accompanied by a massive population explosion, child labour, poverty and destitution were rife. In major cities, half of all infants died from dirt, neglect and infectious diseases such as whooping cough, diphtheria, smallpox and tuberculosis. Older children suffered accidents and abuse in mines, cotton mills and on the streets (Aynsley-Green 2004).

> In 1884 the Liverpool Society for the Protection of Children was formed, subsequently transformed into the National Society for the Prevention of Cruelty to Children. It is noteworthy that the Royal Society for the Prevention of Cruelty to Animals had been founded 60 years earlier in 1824. What does this say about the importance given to children over animals in 19th century England?
>
> (Al Aynsley-Green, National Clinical Director
> for Children, September 2002)

Eventually, the seeds of social reform were sown, as leading figures including Elizabeth Browning, Joseph Rowntree, Bramwell Booth and Dr Barnado spoke out and took action. Great Ormond Street Hospital was born out of the outrage of Charles West and Charles Dickens that England, as the richest and most powerful country in Europe, was also the only country that failed to provide health care for the sick children of the poor.

Is it not outrageous – I use that word deliberately – is it not outrageous that we live in the fourth richest country in the world and still have so many children living in poverty? In Bolton yesterday I was told that 30 per cent or more of the children in that locality live in poverty.

(Al Aynsley Green, National Clinical Director for Children, September 2002)

Despite a further 150 years of progress, by 2001, when Ian Kennedy's report drew attention to the inadequacies in children's health care, all was far from rosy on the broader children's agenda. Inequalities across social groups were widening, with unacceptable numbers of children still living in poverty, an increase in the number of young offenders, an influx of refugee children with unmet health needs and an increase in the number of vulnerable children needing protection. It was in this climate that the death of Victoria Climbié fired a drive for further reform.

The Children's National Service Framework

Three years on, in October 2004, the Department of Health, in partnership with the Department of Education and Skills, released the National Service Framework (NSF) for Children, Young People and Maternity Services (Department of Education and Skills and Department of Health 2004). NSFs are produced by the Government to safeguard the delivery of specific aspects of health care. They do this by setting standards that all health-care organisations have to deliver. For example, the Cancer NSF set a range of targets, which included reducing waiting times to diagnosis and treatment, and cancer services are now judged against those standards.

The Children's NSF is the biggest (weighing in at 2.5 kilogrammes!) and most complex NSF published to date: first, because childhood has its roots in pregnancy, so care has to start with pregnant mothers – and even before that with preconception advice; and second, because the health and well-being of children involves not just the NHS, but also schools, Social Services departments, the voluntary sector and, most importantly, parents and children themselves. The Children's NSF was therefore the culmination of a series of policy documents crossing all the statutory agencies, but it was the Kennedy and the Laming reports that were particularly close to the hearts of those involved in its development. It had an ambitious aim: to produce joined-up, well-coordinated services for children and families that not only provide best possible support for them when they are ill, but also when they are well. Because of this, much of the Children's NSF is about supporting parenting, promoting children's development and empowering children and families to take care of their own health, as well as providing services for children who are ill or who have complex health needs. Overarching these aspirations is a strong intent to reduce inequalities and to ensure that children from disadvantaged backgrounds have the same opportunities to live healthy lives and realise their full potential as their more fortunate peers.

To what extent will this process of reform help Daniel and others like him? There is no doubt that the principles are right: the Children's NSF promotes better networked care, ongoing development of children's trusts, and services designed around the needs of children and families using them, not around the needs of organisations. In other words, it sets out to tackle the very problems described earlier in this chapter: funding disputes and poor communication between organisations, lack of respite care and isolation. At this stage, it is hard to tell how well the Children's NSF will translate in practice, but at its launch, Al Aynsley-Green was clear about one very important point: fine words will only become meaningful if supported by active engagement from those at the front line.

AT THE FRONT LINE: TRUST AND TRANSFERS

When we are ill we want to know that we have a doctor whose technical knowledge and skills we can be sure of, on whose honesty we can rely, and who will treat us empathetically with the respect and courtesy to which we are entitled. We need to be sure that the hospital or primary care team to which our doctor usually belongs works effectively and safely so we can be assured that we are getting good quality care. And we need good access to care.

(Irvine 2003)

Having discussed how the health-care systems could be better stream-lined to improve Daniel's care, what about the people on the front line and their personal role in supporting the Johnson family?

In theory, Susan should have been delighted to be taking Daniel home, once he was well enough to leave the Albion. St Michael's proximity to home would simplify life. If he needed to be admitted again, visits, and looking after Sara, would be easier. Being linked in to the local network would help the family access all sorts of care, such as help and advice from the local physiotherapist about Daniel's treatment and the expertise of the home-care nursing team. And leaving the Albion was a clear sign that Daniel was getting better. Nonetheless, Susan was afraid.

Susan's anxiety stemmed from a lack of trust in the local team; a lack of trust that was not based on experience, but simply on uncertainty about a group of people that she didn't know and who had yet to prove themselves in her eyes.

Trust

Daniel's situation – transferring from highly specialist to local care – was relatively unusual, but many of the fears that this transition raised for his parents are common. For example, the same anxieties beset parents of premature babies as they first move out of the neonatal intensive-care setting, families of children leaving hospital to go home and, indeed, adults transferring out of intensive care, from hospital to home or from one hospital to another. No matter how alien the 'high-tech' environment may have been, familiarity inevitably becomes an anchor, and once that anchor is lifted, families can feel at sea again. They have to transfer their trust to another set of professionals.

The dictionary definition of trust is 'A firm belief that a person or thing can be relied on' ('trust' in Bandolier 2002). Trust is essential in many relationships: between clinicians and patients, between team members, between patients and institutions, between the public and the medical profession. And, of course, the issue of trust between the public and the Government is one that has come under much scrutiny in the past decade. The impact of medical error on trust is discussed further in Chapter 5. Perhaps not surprisingly, studies have shown (Calnan and Sanford 2004) that the public has a lot more confidence in individual doctor–patient relationships than in the health-care system more broadly, and the broader issue of public trust in health-care systems is discussed in Chapter 7. In this chapter, however, we will focus more specifically on trust between the patient and the clinicians or teams directly involved in their care.

There has been relatively little research on the factors that are important in developing trust between patients and clinicians. Such research as there is has focused primarily on trust in the doctor–patient relationship, and this is perhaps a response to the recent high-profile cases already alluded to. More work is needed, not just in looking at this relationship, but equally importantly in looking at trust in nurses, allied health professionals and other clinicians, as they take on much broader roles in patient care.

But does trust really matter, or is this just motherhood and apple pie? A study by Thom et al. (2002) showed that it does matter – not just psychologically, but in real material outcomes. The study showed that patients who had lower trust in their doctors were more likely to report dissatisfaction with the services they received, were less likely to follow the advice given and less likely to report symptom improvement two weeks later, when compared to patients who had higher trust in those same doctors.

Based on the research that we have available, what facets are important in developing trust between doctors and patients? Checkland et al. (2004) suggest that there are two important aspects to developing trust: a more open dialogue with patients and more equality in the balance of power between patients and doctors.

As parents, we started to interpret results, predict ill health before it took hold of our child, and fight madly to get respite for Katie and for us. And to fight for the clinicians to keep us as an inpatient as we did not know what was wrong with our child. And because no one could afford the time to sit and discuss the fact that they did not know, we took the defensive, when all we wanted was communication and some perspective on things.

Whilst at home, I remember that after exhaustive phone calls to both hospitals involved in Katie's care about what we should do regards this or that symptom, I began to feel that the clinicians I was talking to did not care and did not have the answers. This was a very sad place to be.

(Tracey and Keith McBride, parents of a child with complex health needs)

How to achieve trust and a better balance in the relationship between patients and clinicians? The five top ranked behaviours in developing trust in another study by Thom (2001) are shown below:

Box 3.2 Learning points for doctors: behaviours most important for patient trust

1 Being comforting and caring.
2 Demonstrating competency.
3 Encouraging questions and answering clearly.
4 Explaining what the patient needs to know.
5 Referring to another specialist if needed.

(Thom 2001)

It is interesting to see that being comforting and caring is as important as demonstrating competency, and that admitting limitations and referring on to a colleague is likely to increase rather than decrease trust. Whilst medical education continues to focus on ensuring that doctors are competent in diagnosis and treatment, there is now a clear recognition of the importance of teaching young doctors how to communicate in a way that will inspire trust and confidence.

Transfers

The process of transfer of care involves so many people in so many places and requires such attention to detail, that it is easy to see how things frequently go wrong somewhere along the way. For instance, just taking the example of Daniel's home oxygen, Penny would have needed to sort out a plethora of issues. First, she needed to visit the Johnsons' home, to make sure there were no open gas fires, to make sure the house was suitable for the oxygen concentrator, to organise the ordering of back-up oxygen cylinders, to check that they could be carried on his pushchair, to make sure Susan and Matthew were trained in use of the equipment, to make sure that both the insurance company and the fire brigade had been informed that there were oxygen cylinders in the house and, at the same time, to reassure Susan and Matthew that despite all these precautions the whole project was completely safe for them and Daniel.

Systems do not always work perfectly – and there are important lessons to be drawn from the times when things go wrong.

Getting it wrong

Smith and Daughtrey (2000) summarised some of the key messages from families about the pitfalls and problems that they faced when their children were discharged from hospital. Few of the themes involved deficits that needed to be fixed by government directives, additional funding or more staff. They were not rocket science, but things that could be fixed by thinking things through from the patient's perspective.

'The discharge process' was the first stumbling block. If the timing of the discharge was imposed rather than negotiated, or if parents and their child left a little too soon, the stress was enormous:

> I think I worried more that first night, I kept thinking should I have brought him home? Should I have let him stay another night? I was all stressed up about it.
>
> (Smith and Daughtrey 2000: 816)

> At the very end of Katie's life we were expected to be discharged home to the community with the understanding that our local hospital was to be accessed if needed. Katie was obviously too clinically unwell to be going anywhere, and the feeling I have, on reflection, was that there was a pressure for resources (beds) and a lack of a lead clinician during this time. To bring this into context in transfer of care, parents should feel comfortable with the decision of discharge, and it should always be led by a consultant so that the parents can be fully informed, and can argue if they feel discharge is inappropriate.
>
> (Tracey and Keith McBride, parents of a child with complex health needs)

Perhaps the most common theme was 'information, information, information'. Written information, verbal information and information repeated both before and following discharge.

> I would have just liked them to talk to me a bit more and explain
> what to do if she has another fit, because I still don't know what
> to do.
>   I asked the questions at the time but when I got back to my
> room I thought 'I could have asked her this and I could have
> asked her that' . . . and I never got to ask those questions because
> she was busy doing whatever she was doing.
>
> (Smith and Daughtrey 2000: 817)

The need for support and advice at home, as well as in hospital, is
evident from the above quotes. This makes it crucially important that
discharge information gets to the GP and the community team before
the family does. Otherwise, not only are they unable to provide the
support that is desperately needed, but trust in the home team is
undermined because they are, through no fault of their own, ignorant
of the key facts. Once at home, the stress of not knowing who to turn
to for advice is another real burden for families:

> You feel you want to come home and that you'll be better off,
> but there [in hospital] you are surrounded by people who know
> what to do if something goes wrong, but at home you're on your
> own and it's easy to get things out of proportion.
>
> (Smith and Daughtrey 2000: 817)

The first forty-eight hours after discharge seem to be a critical time,
and parents in Smith and Daughtry's study felt particularly anxious if
unsure who to turn to during that period. GPs also felt that the hospital
should maintain some kind of responsibility during that time, perhaps
with a telephone hotline.

Getting it right

Sadly, I feel that the stress we experienced was increased by the poor systems in place. But for us it was also the failings of an individual to make the journey smoother by being a better communicator, explaining more to us and assisting liaison with other departments.

Each professional within a child's ill health has their jobs and boundaries, and some of the needs of children fall in between their remits. If there was a coordinator involved, the transitions could be made more fluid and the liaison, coordination and support would be so valuable. Things should be looked at holistically; maybe there should be more case conferences with clinicians and families on regular basis.

In a way, helping with Snakes and Ladders has meant we have had to relive all those terrible occasions from the past. But if, by documenting them, it means that families and clinicians reading this book will develop a better understanding and come up with better ways of doing things, then it will have been a worthwhile testimony to Katie's memory.

(Tracey McBride, mother of a child with complex health needs)

It is easy to see how practical issues can get in the way of doing things right. Staff sickness, inadequate staffing, wrong addresses on computer systems all contribute. But there is still much that is down to the individual, not the system.

As explained earlier in this chapter, when we played this scenario out on stage at GOSH, we 'did it wrong' and included every possible bungle and failure of communication that can occur along the pathway. Staff found it uncomfortable to watch, because it wasn't an episode of *Fawlty Towers*, which is funny because it is so safely unreal. People squirmed when watching this episode because it was all too real – maybe not every error at once, but far too many for comfort. The following points are crucial in ensuring that the transfer proceeds smoothly, and the principles apply to adult as well as paediatric transfers:

Box 3.3 Learning points for the 'discharging' clinical team: managing transfer of care

- Discuss discharge arrangements carefully with family members.
- Give parents adequate verbal and written information about their child's condition, common complications, treatment, and so on.
- Discuss the roles of GP, CCN, local hospital and tertiary teams in their child's future management. Make sure they know who to contact at primary-, secondary- and tertiary-care levels, and how. If discharging from tertiary care and trying to forge links between families and secondary or primary care, encourage families to contact these in the first instance.
- Arrange for them to meet all relevant professionals within the services that they may need to access, before they need them. Arrange home visits where relevant.
- Pre-empt any likely causes of concern, such as safe and acceptable differences in approach between different services.
- If giving supplies for patients or parents, such as dressings or medication, check they have sufficient short-term supplies and know where to get more as needed.
- Ensure that comprehensive information about patients is provided to other professionals. Telephone communication is important but not sufficient – written information is also needed. This can usefully be dictated in front of parents or patients, questions answered at that time and copies sent on immediately to all parties.
- Make sure families are clear about follow-up plans. Fax discharge summary, follow-up plans and nursing/pharmacy communications to relevant teams on discharge, and ensure that parents receive these promptly.
- Ensure that all those involved in a child's care know who else is involved, and how they can contact each other.

Box 3.4 Learning points for all team members: managing transfer of care

- Demonstrate confidence in colleagues and other individuals and teams.
- Do not try to impose new ways of doing things if the patient or family has a safe and established way that works for them.
- Do not criticise previous care regimes.
- Remember that patients need time to let go of previous relationships, even after transfer, and may initially find it hard to relate to a new set of professionals.
- Be realistic about what the service can provide. For example, resist the temptation to say 'We can do that by next week', when realistically you know it's going to take two to three weeks. If there are going to be delays, let the patient know and explain why.
- Say what you're going to do, and do what you said you would.
- Respect confidentiality. If you have been given information about a patient during transfer, ask permission before passing it on to colleagues.

As a patient, you may feel like a passive partner in this transfer, at the mercy of whether or not your care is handed over to a clinician or team that you consider 'trustworthy'. To some extent this may be true, since choices for local care are necessarily limited, despite efforts to increase specific aspects of patient choice. However, there are some pointers worth remembering:

Box 3.5 Learning points for patients and families: developing trust during transfers

The following points apply whether you are a patient yourself or are the carer of a child or relative.

- Your new team may do things differently. Different is just that – it is not necessarily better or worse.

---

continued

- Remember that the receiving clinician may be just as nervous about meeting an 'expert patient' as you are about having to forge a new relationship.
- Provided you are happy to have copies of letters about your care or that of your child, ask the hospital or team you are leaving for the most up-to-date correspondence and summaries.
- The 'constant' during this transfer is you and your family. Do not be afraid to speak up if you think the receiving team has incorrect or out-of-date information.
- Acknowledging your anxiety about the new situation can be helpful. It will give the receiving team the chance to talk you through the local systems and to address any particular concerns that you may flag up.

Finally, there are some very important practical issues about 'taking control' and staying on top of some of the organisational demands and complexities of managing a chronic illness.

Box 3.6 Learning points for patients and families: taking control

The following points apply, whether you are a patient yourself or are the carer of a child or relative.

- You now have a right to be asked whether you wish to receive copies of correspondence written about you or your child by health professionals. If you are not automatically copied in to letters, you should feel free to request this (see Department of Health Guidance on copying letters, on <http://www.dh.gov.uk>).
- As time goes by, you will have many letters, reports, etc. A bit of organisation at the beginning (perhaps before you realise how many there will be) will help enormously in the long run. Buy an A4 file and dividers, and file letters according to specialty or hospital, as they come in.

- Many hospitals operate a 'Shared Care File' to promote good communication between all health professionals. Suggest this if you feel it would help.
- If your child has numerous admissions or if you simply want to keep track of all the appointments, get and keep a diary just for that child. Note 'good' days and 'poorly' days, and GP and all other appointments. This will give you a very good background to keep abreast of any future developments – one day or one week can merge into the next when you are busy and tired.
- Keep a file for state benefits; remember that your child may be eligible for Disability Living Allowance and you may be entitled to Carer's Allowance. Ensure that you apply as soon as possible, as it is only payable from the date the application is received. Again, keep copies of all correspondence.
- Holidays and insurance may prove to be problematic if your child has a medical condition. There are companies that specialise in this area and many of the high-street insurers will provide insurance after a medical questionnaire has been completed. Either Contact A Family <http://www.cafamily.org.uk> or many of the other voluntary organisations keep details.
- Get in touch with any of the specialist medical charities: many have support groups and key workers who can provide a wealth of practical experience and support to children and their families with a new diagnosis.

At the end of the day

Jack Stebbing pulled up in the practice car park, grabbed the remains of his half-eaten sandwich from the passenger seat and dictated a brief referral letter about the patient he had just seen on a home visit as he walked through the back door of the surgery into the kitchen area. Pausing only to pour a hasty cup of coffee and to drop the dictaphone tape in to his secretary, he arrived at the practice meeting just ten minutes late.

It was almost full house. Mary, the senior partner, was away, but Nancy and David, the two other partners, were both there, along with Sally, the practice nurse. They were all involved in an animated argument about an ex-heroin addict who was now on methadone maintenance treatment. Apparently he had been verbally abusive in the waiting area, calling the receptionist a 'Paki bastard' and overturning a couple of chairs. No one had been hurt, but the new receptionist was pretty shaken.

'Come on, Nancy, you can't save the world,' David said. 'We warned him the last time that we'd remove him from the list if this happened again. How many more times are you going to intervene for him?'

Sally was flicking through a report on the last two incidents. 'Nancy, I do think David's right,' she said. 'I don't think we can carry on putting the reception staff through this.'

Jack had a view, but decided to use the interval to catch his breath and eat the rest of his sandwich rather than getting involved. At that moment the door opened and Penny arrived. Sometimes they didn't see Penny for months, and then they had a run of children under the paediatric home-care team. They were in the middle of just such a run.

'Hi Penny,' Jack said, getting up and pulling a chair forward for her. 'Do come in. I think there are a couple of yours that we need to talk about aren't there? We won't be long. Coffee?'

By the time he returned with a coffee for Penny, he was amazed to discover that Nancy had got her way yet again and had bought just one more chance for her young addict.

Penny brought them quickly up to date on the state of play with Daniel Johnson, who had been discharged from the Albion three months back, and who had recently been in St Michael's with an episode of pneumonia. He was now back home and doing well. She gave a quick rundown on how he was progressing with his oxygen dependence, which was apparently reducing. Her main worry was that the whole family seemed pretty exhausted, and she mentioned that Susan was going to bring Sara in to see Jack, because she'd started complaining of tummy aches, and had missed quite a lot of school. Penny reckoned this was going to turn out to be psychological – a case of school refusal rather than a physical problem – but she was keen to see what Jack thought.

Pulling out another sheaf of notes, she said, 'The other patient I wanted to talk about is Siobhan Macklin. She was a twenty-five-weeker.[1] She's now sixteen weeks old and is being discharged from St Mike's on

---

1 Baby born prematurely at twenty-five weeks gestation (that is, about fifteen weeks early).

Tuesday. Mary came to the discharge-planning meeting, because the family is on her list, but I gather she's away this week, so I said I'd fill everyone in.'

'That's helpful – thanks Penny,' Jack said. Mary, the senior partner, was enjoying a well-earned four-week cruise to celebrate her twentieth wedding anniversary, and everyone was working hard to cover her patients.

'Well, it's an awful story! The mother is only fifteen and a half years old herself and got pregnant after a one-night stand. She was too scared to tell her parents – they're a Catholic family – so she kept it secret. She eventually told one of the counsellors at school and said she wanted an abortion – by which time it was too late. Anyway, a couple of days later, she was out late with a crowd of friends and came off the back of a moped. Just cuts and bruises, but went into premature labour. When she got up to St Mike's, she didn't tell anyone that she was pregnant or that she had labour pains . . . and then by the time they realised what was going on, she ended up delivering on an A&E trolley, with no paediatrician in sight. Upshot was a really delayed resuscitation.'

'What a nightmare for the poor family,' said Nancy. 'How's the baby?'

'Not good,' Penny handed her a copy of the notes she had taken at the discharge planning meeting. 'She had a grade IV bleed.[2] She's clearly going to have really severe spasticity and, sadly, they think she's got very little vision or hearing. Feeding is a terrible struggle at the moment – she takes about an hour for each feed. Oh, and she has pretty bad fits.'

There was a heavy silence. 'Did anyone discuss the possibility of withholding treatment?' David said eventually.

'Well, actually, I did have a cup of coffee with Margaret after the discharge-planning meeting. She's one of the neonatal ward sisters. She told me Siobhan got a bad infection at about twelve weeks, and they talked then about not resuscitating her if she stopped breathing. The thing is, it split the neonatal unit. Half the staff wanted to pull out, and the rest said no.'

'What about her mum?' Sally said. 'We keep talking about the team, but did anyone discuss the options with her or her parents? How were they coping? You said they were devout Catholics?'

'I'm sorry, I'm afraid I don't know. I'm not sure if they asked her or not. Everyone was so distressed about it that I didn't manage to get any more of the details. I would guess that if they had asked her she'd have said to

2 The most severe kind of brain haemorrhage in premature babies – and a particular risk in very small babies, especially if resuscitation is delayed or difficult. Results in very severe disability.

stop treatment. But then she's just a child herself. Maybe they asked her parents – and they may well have said carry on. Who knows?'

'But this kid's life – I mean the mum's life – is going to be completely consumed now, looking after this desperately sick baby,' David said, voicing what they all knew. 'I mean, fair enough, if she'd been a precious baby of a forty-year-old on her third run of IVF.[3] Apart from anything else, she'd probably be the kind who could afford a nanny to look after the child.'

'David, that's outrageous! I don't know how you can say that,' Nancy cut in. 'If you start making judgements about whether a baby should survive based on the social circumstances of the parents, you might as well revert to the Third Reich.'

Penny decided to try to cut into this before things got out of hand. 'The other thing that Margaret told me was that the pro-life lobby on the neonatal unit said that it was wrong to pull out because you couldn't start playing God.'

'That's all very well, but they started playing God the moment they resuscitated this baby in casualty. I don't think you can then put your hands up, call pax and stop playing God just because it's no longer an easy game.' David looked across at Nancy, daring her to challenge him.

UNRESOLVED QUESTIONS: THE RIGHT TO LIFE

We hold these truths to be self evident: that all men are created equal; that they are endowed by their Creator with certain inalienable rights; that amongst these are life, liberty and the pursuit of happiness.

(American Declaration of Independence, 4 July 1776)

---

3 In-vitro fertilisation: the technique used for treating infertility. Babies born by IVF are otherwise known as 'test-tube babies'.

Throughout this chapter we have discussed the burden of caring for a child with complex health needs at home, the strain on the family and the broader issues of how we value children in our society. All of these issues are brought into sharper focus in situations where the disability is greater, and where parents and health-care staff are faced with life and death decisions.

It goes without saying that life and death decisions evoke strong feelings in all concerned – and the ethical issues raised through the above scenario are many and complex. Situations such as the one depicted in our fictitious GP practice are increasingly common as medical advances push the boundaries of doctors' ability to maintain life. The Human Rights Act 1998 provides protection of life and protection from degrading treatment. However, the balance between such rights is often unclear and controversial. Guidance has been developed by the British Medical Association (2001) and the Royal College of Paediatrics and Child Health (1997), and the issue has been debated in court on a number of occasions recently. When it comes to the question raised by this scenario about 'withdrawing', there are three broad issues to consider. What is the basis for such as decision? Who makes the decision? and How is it implemented?

The basis of the decision

There are a number of ways of thinking about the basis of the decision itself – some people find it useful to look at principles of moral philosophy, many rely on religious principles and others on their own 'gut feelings'. What is clear, however, is that analysing each individual case from different perspectives highlights and depersonalises what is often a very difficult decision. Where would these analyses lead us for Siobhan?

David is looking at the consequences or outcome of keeping Siobhan alive, weighing the costs to the family and society as a whole. Such an approach is often termed 'Utilitarian' or 'Consequentialist'. In his eyes, Siobhan will have a life full of medical interventions that will cause her discomfort and often pain. She will have little or no 'happiness'. Her mother, still a child herself, will spend much of her time trying to care for Siobhan. David might also be considering the scarcity of beds, and the fact that by keeping Siobhan in intensive care, many other children who could make a complete recovery may be denied a bed. For David, therefore, the best way forward, looking at 'the greatest happiness for the greatest number', would be to discuss withholding treatment and letting nature take its course.

By contrast, Nancy feels that it is deeply wrong to look at the big picture and not the individual. In her eyes, some things must be protected absolutely and the 'right to life' is one such that must trump all. Although some philosophers have argued that an individual needs to be competent to exercise a right, most people instinctively feel that rights, by their very nature, are intended to protect those least able to speak for themselves. This is reflected in law in Article 2 of the Human Rights Act:

> Everyone's right to life shall be protected by law. No one shall be deprived of his life intentionally, save in the execution of a sentence of a court following his conviction of a crime for which this penalty is provided by law.
>
> (Article 2, Human Rights Act 1998)

Indeed, for those of strong religious faith, the belief that life has an objective intrinsic value based on the sanctity of God's creation means that human life, in whatever form, is sacred and must be protected. As devout Catholics, Siobhan's family may well believe that withdrawing support is deeply morally wrong and that our society must protect individual life at all costs.

However, there is a counter-argument to maintaining life at all costs in Article 3 of the Human Rights Act.

> No one shall be subjected to torture or to inhuman or degrading treatment or punishment.
>
> (Article 3, Human Rights Act 1998)

Does maintaining life at all costs on a ventilator amount to degrading treatment, and how are these rights to be balanced? These complicated questions have been discussed in the courts in a number of cases. What is clear is that each right carries with it a corollary duty, and that every doctor owes a duty to his patients to care for them in their best interests and to do no harm. So which would be the greater harm – withdrawing treatment or maintaining life at all costs?

In balancing the issues, a court will look at what is in the child's best interests. In complicated family scenarios such as this, it is often easy to forget that it is Siobhan, the baby, who is in fact the patient. It is therefore the Children Act 1989 which provides the strongest guidance.

> The child's welfare shall be the paramount consideration.
>
> (Children Act 1989)

Siobhan is going to be severely paralysed, severely intellectually disabled, blind and deaf. She will almost inevitably need to be fed by a gastrostomy (a tube directly into the stomach) and she will have severe seizures. In some instances, there is a 'no purpose' justification for withdrawing treatment; this is based on the judgement that the degree of physical or mental impairment will be so great that it is unreasonable to expect the child to bear it, and that he or she will never be capable of taking part in any self-directed activity. If, in Siobhan's case, her quality of life is going to be so poor, and the pain and discomfort so great, that prolonging her life will not confer net benefit over harm, then continuing burdensome or futile treatment would not be considered to be in her best interests. However, this does raise controversial issues around the valuing of people with disabilities and would not be universally accepted as a justification for withdrawing treatment.

Who makes the decision?

How are these decisions made in reality? In most cases, clinicians and parents are able to discuss the options available together, reaching a common consensus on the best way forward for the child. In such discussions, it is worth remembering that other cultures may support a different way of decision-making. For example, one nurse told the story of how the clinical team thought the parents of a Chinese baby were distant and uninvolved. Once the matter had been openly discussed, it turned out that their culture prohibited them from making any decision about their child. It was the grandparents who had the power to do this, and they had never been invited by the hospital to come to meetings. It is also worth remembering that a conversation about withdrawing treatment, which may have become all too commonplace for the medical team, will be one of the worst times of the family's life. Discussions mentioning medical terms such as 'DNARs' (Do Not Attempt Resuscitation orders), 'pulling out' or 'letting him declare himself' may mean nothing to parents and can only serve to alienate a family that may already feel disempowered, vulnerable and traumatised.

If it becomes impossible to reach agreement, the court has the ultimate decision-making jurisdiction. Over the years, there have been a number of high-profile cases where the team and the family have been unable to reach a decision, and where the court's ruling has been sought. Indeed, the European Court of Human Rights ruled that failure to bring a dispute between a child's family and the treating team before the court is a breach of the child's right to respect for private and family life, protected under Article 8 of the Human Rights Act (*Glass* v. *United Kingdom* [2004] ECHR 61827/00).

The most recent such dispute to attract media attention was the legal battle between Portsmouth Hospital and the parents of Charlotte Wyatt, who was born three months prematurely and who suffered severe damage to her brain and vital organs. Despite her parents' wish to use all possible means to prolong her life, the court ruled that it would not be in Charlotte's best interests to ventilate her if she developed breathing difficulties. The court also confirmed that no clinician can be made to treat a child against what they perceive to be their best interests (*Portsmouth NHS Trust* v. *Wyatt and Ors* [2004] EWHC 2247).

Finally, many hospitals now have clinical ethics committees, which may be able to provide support by giving an objective perspective, although they do not hold any prescriptive power over the final decision.

How should the decision be implemented?

Even had a decision been made to withdraw treatment, the final complexity comes in deciding how this should be done. The courts have made it clear that any action intentionally taken by doctors to bring about death is illegal and murder. However, they have recognised the strange disparity between acts and omissions – the difference between withdrawing or withholding treatment and taking active steps to end someone's life.

If Siobhan was on life support, the team could lawfully withdraw this. If, however, she was breathing independently, the option not to treat a serious infection with antibiotics or to resuscitate her if she had a respiratory arrest would be another way in which this decision might be implemented. Doctors may also find that by administering palliative care (such as morphine) they will end up hastening death and shortening the patient's life. The courts have made it very clear that this practice (often referred to as the doctrine of double effect because one action has two effects) is *only* lawful if the doctor's intention is not to hasten death, but simply to relieve suffering. The fact that death may be precipitated must be an incidental, albeit recognised, side effect.

Perhaps the most difficult moral issues arise in relation to the withdrawal of artificial feeding. This question came before the House of Lords in the landmark case of Tony Bland, the young man tragically left in PVS (persistent vegetative state) following the Hillsborough Football stadium disaster in April 1989 (*Airedale NHS Trust v. Bland* [1983] 1 All ER 821). The court felt that it was lawful to withdraw ANH (artificial nutrition and hydration) given that Bland was insensate and thus could gain no benefit from such treatment, rendering it 'futile'. ANH was seen as medical treatment, which could therefore be withdrawn. This definition of ANH as medical treatment and not basic medical care has been criticised by many as morally unsound. The ramifications of the decision to patients like Siobhan who, although profoundly disabled, are not in PVS have not yet had to be explored by the courts. However, given the rapid advances in neonatal care, and the increasing complexity of the ethical dilemmas that we all face, it is probably only a matter of time before the courts will have to address such issues.

4 No room at the inn

Easy rider

Susan pressed the off switch on the TV remote control and the living room was quiet for the first time all day. She wondered why they'd watched, or half-watched, yet another documentary about the state of the NHS, rather than enjoying some peace and quiet. She stretched out and yawned.

'Isn't it weird? You hear all this stuff all the time about trolley waits in casualty and people waiting years for hip replacements, but we've been really lucky with St Mike's and Dr Stebbing and everyone. Do you think our team is unusual? Or maybe they just pull out all the stops for children?'

Matthew was heading for the kitchen. He'd finally got Daniel through bath, supper and bed and wasn't due to collect Sara from her school disco for another hour. Cystic fibrosis or no cystic fibrosis, prising a six-year-old away from friends, television or any other excuse and pointing him in the general direction of bed was no picnic. Matt was feeling distinctly frayed, but was not about to admit that to Susan.

Over the past three years, since things had been on a more even keel with Daniel, Susan had been doing really well at work. She had progressed from her secretarial job, and had spent six months as an office manager before moving to her latest post, managing the sales department in a local software company. A year ago she had decided to do a BA in management studies through the Open University. Matthew worried about the extra hours of study she had to put in after a hard day at work and was very doubtful that she would be able to see it through. But he was certainly not going to say that to her and was doing his best to support her by doing his fair share with Daniel and around the house. Still, it was a bit galling that Susan seemed to be able to get Daniel to bed in half the time it took him. Matthew knew he was a bit of a soft touch.

'It's true, we've had an easy ride with him these past few years,' he replied, pausing in the doorway. Then, remembering in more detail

Daniel's numerous admissions with chest infections and feeding problems, he thought again. His ideas about what constituted normal family life and an 'easy' time had gradually shifted to accommodate chronic illness. 'Well, not exactly easy when you think how often he's been in St Mike's. And he's not been in great form these past few weeks. But I guess you're right – St Mike's have always been really good with him.'

Susan thought back to the first admission to St Michael's, and to how petrified she'd been that they wouldn't be able to cope. Over the years, when they'd been in and out of Rainbow Ward with Daniel, she had seen some very sick children being managed by the team, and she was amazed at how they did so well with such a diverse range of problems and so few staff. Daniel was due to be admitted to the Albion the following week to have some investigations done, and, ironically, she felt rather unsettled by it. Although they still went up to the Albion for outpatient appointments between visits to St Michael's, it was years since Daniel had actually had to be admitted there. She had asked Dr Khan why it couldn't all be sorted out at St Michael's. But Dr Khan had been insistent that these were specialist tests to see why Daniel was having so much trouble with vomiting after meals, and why he'd had such a run of chest infections in the past few months. So Susan had accepted that there was no alternative.

And so to beds

Peter Soames was having one of those days. The lot of a bed manager was not always a happy one, he reflected. As he put the phone down after talking to one of the clinical site practitioners – the Albion's small pool of very senior nurses who took overall charge of the hospital by day and night – he looked gloomily at the lengthening list of bed problems. Two closed on Starlight Ward due to large overspends and overactivity in that department. Cherry Ward not taking any admissions because of an outbreak of diarrhoea and vomiting. The problems generated because of the child who had come into Douglas Ward for overnight tests and was still there seven days later due to complications; this meant that several children booked in for tests over the following few days had needed to be booked elsewhere or cancelled. And now he had just been told that they needed to use the last bed on Neptune for an incoming renal patient, so things were getting tighter by the minute.

The most immediate problem was to locate a bed for a transfer from A&E in Barnet for a child with serious head injuries who had fallen out of a tree house. The neurosurgical registrar was waiting anxiously on this one, because the child needed surgery as quickly as possible.

As he reached for the phone to call one of his diminishing list of possible wards, it rang again: 'Is that the bed manager?'

'Yes . . . this is Peter. Peter Soames. Who's calling?' He couldn't believe his bad luck, as it became apparent that it was the mother of a child who had been booked for investigation on Douglas Ward. It wasn't his job to talk directly to patients or families, but there was no way he could stop Mrs Johnson as she launched into a tirade about how her son had been due in that morning for two or three days, for tests, and she'd just got into work to find a message left on the answerphone yesterday evening about a bed problem – meaning there wasn't a place for him. He could see how this had happened. Someone cancelling the admissions had obviously mistaken her work number for her home number and had left the message on the wrong phone. He had to concede that finding her way through to the bed manager was not only logical but also a great achievement. But he needed to get rid of her and sort out this Barnet problem.

'Errr, Mrs Johns—, Mrs . . . I'm terribly sorry, I really can't help you. You need to go through the ward sister . . . You can't reach her? Oh, I see, she's on a course? . . . The nurse covering doesn't know? . . . OK . . .' He was beginning to feel sorry for her, but had to stick to his guns, 'I'll see what I can do, but I can't promise anything. I'm sorry. You might need to wait until tomorrow . . . Oh, I see, Daniel's not eaten since last night to get ready for the tests today . . . he's on his way with his father to the train. Well, can you reach them, tell them not to come just yet? Maybe if he has a meal now . . . we haven't got beds available,' he said, praying silently he'd find one for the critical kid in Barnet, 'but I'll call some wards and ask them to get back to you if they have a bed . . .' Would he? Would he find time?

'Oakshott Ward? Peter Soames here. Look, I've got a kid needs to come in from Barnet. He's four. Fell out of a treehouse. The neurosurgeons need to get him to theatre fast. Can you take him? . . . You might be able to later? Well, how much later? He's not got much time to hang around by the sound of it. Oh right. You're waiting for someone to go home, but the ambulance hasn't turned up to get her? Well, will she go today for sure? Can I tell the Barnet team to start travelling? . . . It's too risky . . . why? Oh right, you've half promised the bed for a child who may come back from intensive care today, and you won't know until after the intensive care ward round? Yes, of course it's understandable . . .'

'Barry Ward? Yes, it's me. Yes, I'm after a bed. . . . Well, if you've got one but you're keeping it free for an emergency, I've got the perfect emergency for you. Can I get him on his way from Barnet . . . it sounds bad . . . Great. Great. Thanks.'

The phone rang again before Peter could pick it up to call Barnet. It was the A&E sister there. She sounded upset. 'Mr Soames? It's Nell Grieves.

Look, don't worry about trying to find a bed for our transfer. He's . . .,'
she stopped in mid-sentence, '. . . well, it's too late now.'

Peter wanted to give a moment's thought to the child. To a family
somewhere in North London whose little boy had just died. But there wasn't
time. He picked up the phone and got straight back on to Barry Ward.

'Hi. Me again. Look, forget about the Barnet boy . . .' [Christ, that
sounds terrible; how can I be so matter of fact?] Can you take a kid in for
a couple of days for tests? Cystic fibrosis boy. Needs admission today –
got tests booked for this afternoon.' As he said it, Peter hoped against hope
that it wasn't too late to get back to Mrs Johnson and tell her that Daniel
should still get the train, shouldn't have breakfast. The sister had asked a
question, 'Will he have a Portacath?' 'Dunno – probably, possibly. Why?
. . . Not sure you've got anyone who can use it? But . . . you're all trained
nurses aren't you?'

Portacaths, implanted devices that allow easy access to the bloodstream
for giving drugs and taking tests, weren't that uncommon, yet this was
the second time since he'd joined the Albion that Peter had heard this
one, and it appalled him. He knew that at Fettsham General, where he'd
worked for five years before joining the Albion, the paediatric nurses
couldn't be so precious; with just one children's ward, they had to get on
and cope.

But back there he'd heard variations on exactly the same theme
with adult patients: nurses on the general surgery ward telling him they
couldn't care for a neurosurgery patient, nurses on the chest ward saying
they couldn't manage a patient with failing kidneys. And if a patient had
severe mental-health problems or a learning disability, it was a complete
nightmare getting a ward to look after them when they had other health
problems.

Last time this had happened at the Albion he'd intended to raise it with
his manager, but it had got lost among more pressing concerns. This time,
as he put the phone down, he tore a yellow sticky off the pad on his desk,
scribbled 'Too specialised to care?', had a brief misgiving that he'd not
remember what it meant and stuck it on his computer where he'd at least
see it.

Peter tried three more wards. The first had lots of beds – a brief ray of
hope – but they also had four high-dependency patients and were short-
staffed so couldn't take any more. No way. The next could offer a bed,
but only for twenty-four hours. He knew the Johnson child needed to be in
for two days, so that was no good. But it definitely warranted another
prominently placed yellow sticky – 'BED!!!!!!!! Briony Ward' – someone
would need it as the day wore on, for sure. Among his last hopes was
Prior Ward.

'What d'you mean it's the wrong day to call?!' He knew, but pretended incredulity at the comment, his tiny attempt to get back at them for the frustration it caused him.

'Oh, I see,' he said, sarcasm heavy in his voice, 'It's your doctors' clinic day and you need to keep beds free just in case they want to admit someone?'

He hung up. There was no fighting this one. Earmarking beds and other bed-blocking tactics was a luxury the hospital could ill afford, but it was apparently a tradition that wouldn't change imminently. But at least the consultant who was the worst offender on Prior Ward was retiring at Christmas, so it was easiest just to wait for him to go.

When Peter located an empty bed on Davenport Ward but was told it couldn't be used yet as the cleaners were too busy to sort out the cubicle,[1] he finally lost it with Millie, the ward sister. 'Fine,' he snapped, 'I'll come up and clean it myself – aren't they trying to encourage NHS staff to work across boundaries?' and banged the phone down.

Two minutes later, Millie rang back and told him to get the Johnsons in – she'd sort it somehow, so could he just call the family?

Peter felt guilty about having shouted at her. He knew she was under just as much pressure as he was, and he normally got on well with her; they even had a laugh. He ripped another sticky label off his pad, wrote on it 'Thanks and sorry card to Millie on Davenport', and added it to the army of yellow squares that was fast massing to cover his computer screen.

Matthew blue

Matthew was outside Davenport Ward, on the payphone to his mother, Bridget.

'It's just nonsense. We ended up coming in to a different ward, and even when we got here the bed wasn't ready. Then in the complete muddle Daniel missed his slot, so he didn't get this special X-ray thing till now, and then only because some other kid didn't turn up. And his cubicle . . . it's filthy, though there's a mop in the corner and some bloke in a tie said he'd be back later to clean it, which seemed a bit improbable.'

'Oh, Matthew. It's really tough for you isn't it? How's Susan?'

'She's at home, and is trying to sort out someone to drop in on Sara so that she can get down to stay with Daniel tonight. Of course, Sara's old enough to stay alone and doesn't need it, but I've got to get back for a

---

1 Single-bedded room, used if patients are either infectious or vulnerable to infection.

night shift, and Susan worries about her being in the house on her own when neither of us can be phoned if there's a problem. It was all true, what they said about it being easier to sort out Daniel's treatment at St Michael's. Coming in here has been a real nightmare.'

Matthew's parents lived in Edinburgh and, though they got down when they could, Bridget still felt badly that it wasn't often enough. She felt it especially acutely now. Wished she could help her son more.

'Anyway,' Matthew said, sounding resigned, 'at least we're here now, and I guess it's the right place. It's hard though, Mum. Susan told me Sara was really upset when she got home from school and Daniel wasn't there. She'd forgotten he was coming here. And then she got really cross when Susan said she'd have to come here tonight, and Susan was angry with Sara for not asking anything about Daniel and about the tests or about how things were going. And apparently all Sara said was "Of course I want to know how things are going. I want to know when someone's going to sort him out properly so we can get our lives back." Anyway, it all escalated, and Susan called Sara a selfish little cow, and now they're both really upset.'

Bridget couldn't find anything to say. She'd grown fond of Sara and was sure she'd been upset at herself for forgetting about Daniel's tests, angry with no one and everyone about the disruption, and mainly just wanted her parents and little brother back to being OK.

Cut! Rewind

The Johnsons had shifted their trust from the Albion to St Michael's, and things had been going well there. They had understood that this was no 'downgrade' but a sensible step towards improving care for their son and towards making life easier for all of them. They had developed a great deal of confidence in their local services. Now they had to accept that Daniel needed to go back to the Albion, and that this was the right thing and no reflection against St Michael's. And, yet again, circumstances had conspired against them, and they had had a stressful admission. They had watched enough television, read enough articles and had enough conversations to know the philosophy: the NHS Plan sets out a new relationship with patients and families, shaping treatment around their needs and lives. To some extent, they were sold on the theory, but somehow it didn't always seem to work out that way in practice.

By contrast, to Peter Soames, the basic problem of his day looked simple: not enough beds. If only the Albion had more beds, maybe Peter's life would be a lot easier and so would that of the Johnsons. But underlying this apparently straightforward solution is a complex web of resource and staffing issues that sits at the heart of much of the political discontent surrounding today's NHS. In resource terms, a 'bed' for Daniel actually means a ward with enough nursing staff, the relevant doctors, the ward clerk, the cleaning staff, catering department, the ward pharmacist, the IT support staff, the medical secretary, Peter Soames managing the beds, the X-ray department doctors, nurses and administrative staff . . . the list is endless. If Daniel's entire pathway from admission to discharge were tracked, it is probable that at least 100 staff would make some contribution to his stay. And that's before considering the 'non-staff' costs: the drugs, the food, the laundry costs, replacement costs for the X-ray equipment, and so on.

So to generate more beds means more staff, and more staff means more money. Politicians have acknowledged that there has been long-standing underinvestment in the NHS, but would putting more money in the system have ensured that Daniel had a bed? What about the other complexities, such as how to recruit and retain staff in areas where they can't afford to live. And how to manage when there just aren't enough staff to recruit, because there are national shortages of some professional groups?

Was there a bed problem at the Albion because too few staff were juggling too few resources, or could things have been managed better? Perhaps there could have been better joint-working, staff working differently or better prioritisation of resources? To what extent was the health-care system to blame, and how much could those at the front line have influenced the outcome?

Readers may feel that these problems should be addressed by those charged with delivering and managing health services. But with the emphasis on patient choice and user involvement, the public needs to be informed and involved. The issues may be complex and difficult, but they need to be transparent to all, because, as is explained at the end of this chapter, patients and users are increasingly being expected to contribute to decisions about best use of available resources, as well as making informed decisions about their own care.

THE HEALTH-CARE SYSTEM: UNDERSTANDING WORKFORCE ISSUES

> In the end, the NHS is the people who work for it.
>
> (Alan Milburn, 2 July 2002)

If the Chancellor of the Exchequer, in a moment of unparalleled generosity, were to write a blank cheque for the NHS, would all its problems be solved? The simple answer is that whilst this would have a hugely positive impact, there would still be major problems in training, recruiting and retaining enough staff. And the issue is not just about numbers, but about the right staff doing the right jobs in the right place at the right time. So it would seem that to understand the problems of finding a bed for Daniel, we have to know more about the issues affecting the NHS workforce.

Is there a health-care professional in the house?

Health care is a labour-intensive business involving an estimated 35 million employees worldwide (Geneva International Labour Office 1999). The NHS currently employs well over one million staff and faces ongoing challenges in recruiting and retaining enough employees to cope with the health-care needs of the population. How have we arrived at this problem?

> The NHS employs 386,000 nurses – about the same as the population of Bristol. Its doctors (109,000) outnumber the population of Scarborough (106,700). Its scientists and therapists (122,100) are more numerous than the people of Norwich (121,600).
>
> (Carvel 2004)

Worldwide, there has been a long-standing shortfall of health-care staff, although some prefer to talk about a global 'imbalance of supply'. In response to the demand for health-care professionals, the developing countries have gradually become net exporters of trained staff, with migration really gaining momentum in the 1960s. The issue was brought to public attention when a survey demonstrated that in 1972 alone there was a net loss of physicians from developing countries of 52,800, and a net gain to developed countries of 65,700, mainly to the USA and United Kingdom. This represented a staggering 8.5 per cent of the physician stock of the developing countries (Martineau, Decker and Bundred 2002). By the mid-1970s, 35 per cent of all hospital physicians in the United Kingdom were trained overseas, 60 per cent of them in developing countries. Many of them were working in 'less desirable' posts that had been left unfilled by British doctors because they did not have training or teaching-hospital status. At the same time, it was estimated that about 135,000 nurses (or 4 per cent of the world total) were outside their country of birth or training, and more Filipino nurses were registered in the USA and Canada than in the Philippines (Martineau, Decker and Bundred 2002).

By the early 1970s, policy-makers were starting to worry about the impact on the developing world and to recognise that this was not an acceptable way to staff our own health services. There had to be a way of putting brakes on the 'brain drain' from developing countries, and ideas such as compensating them for their investment in training were mooted. However, despite these good intentions, the United Kingdom has continued to rely on overseas staff to support the NHS and today we are still dealing with major workforce deficits, more than thirty years on from the original discussions. The NHS Plan (NHS Executive 2000) was explicit about the problems of staffing the NHS. Its promise of 7,500 more consultants, 2,000 more GPs, 20,000 extra nurses and 6,500 extra therapists by 2004 has been one of the most widely publicised government pledges, alongside a commitment to increased investment. The identified staffing shortfalls apply right across the workforce, not only to professional staff such as nurses, doctors, pharmacists, physiotherapists, radiographers, and so on, but also to all the non-professional support staff who are essential to the smooth running of the service. Moving patients in and out of beds is like a carefully choreographed dance; even one missing dancer leaves a glaring gap. Peter Soames's search for beds was frustrated by so many problems; the cleaner who was not available to prepare a cubicle for a new patient and the ambulance driver who was not available to take a child home left gaps that were as important as the shortage of nurses.

So why has staffing the NHS been such an insoluble problem? Why are we still partially dependent on overseas recruitment to run our health service, and what other measures have been put in place to support the Government's pledges? Some of the problems inherent in the planning process are outlined below, as well as the steps being taken to remedy these deficits:

Problems in workforce planning

It would seem a self-evident truth that any organisation training nearly 5000 people a year and employing nearly 100,000 highly trained specialists, would have a sophisticated mechanism for predicting future needs and possible excesses or shortfalls, and for deciding numbers of new trainees [. . .] Needless to say, the NHS has almost no such mechanisms in place.

(Kitson, McManus and Pringle 1996: 106)

Balancing supply and demand of health-care professionals is a complex task, with no easy recipe for success. Those most closely involved in workforce planning would be the first to admit that it operates on a 'boom and bust' cycle, and the only certainty is of getting it wrong. It is easy to see why this should be the case. Simplistic predictions based on input–output equations can easily overestimate the number of health-care professionals being 'fed' into the system from training institutions. Training places are reduced but, meanwhile, new social and economic trends result in a loss of health-care staff from the workforce. These include staff of both sexes choosing to work part-time or to take career breaks; the cost of living, especially in larger cities; the poor status and pay of some health-care roles; and increasing global mobility. So despite training what seems to be the right number of staff, shortages continue to be a constant problem.

Matters took a turn for the worse in the early 1990s when, as part of the NHS reforms and the introduction of the internal market, the responsibility for commissioning education of many key professional groups was decentralised and became employer-led. NHS trusts and other local stakeholders could not possibly provide the necessary perspective to anticipate the demands of changing models of care and broader national employment trends. Workforce-planning in nursing was particularly badly affected, with a dramatic drop in the number of nurses in training in England from 75,000 in 1984 to less than half that number by 1994. In 1994–5, the Department of Health implemented a sharp U-turn, and student places have since been increased year on year. Whilst the strategy is right, the system is creaking at the edges in trying to accommodate the huge numbers of trainee nurses. Pressure on both the higher-education institutions and the hospitals in which students need training placements is unprecedented.

Planning of the medical workforce is just as problematic. Data from the Organisation for Economic Cooperation and Development (OECD) demonstrated that in 1960 the number of doctors per capita of the population was fairly uniform between the OECD countries at around 1,000 per million (Scherer 2004). A large gap then opened, and those countries that adopted a policy of regulating medical-school intake (including the United Kingdom, Japan, Canada and New Zealand) now have relatively low numbers of doctors per capita (approximately 2,000 per million) and have had to turn to foreign suppliers to compensate for underinvestment. By contrast, those countries that did not adopt this policy (including Belgium, Greece, Austria and Switzerland) have had substantial growth and now have ratios of 3,500–4,500 per million. In fact, the United Kingdom now has the dubious distinction of having a lower doctor–patient ratio than Canada, America, Australia, New Zealand or any other country in Europe.

Other very specific characteristics of the workforce need to be taken into account. For example, the NHS nursing workforce is ageing, with proportionately more nurses in their fifties in this decade than in the past decade (Buchan and Edwards 2000: 1067). In addition, the Asian doctors who arrived in the United Kingdom in the 1960s and 1970s, and who have been a crucial part of the GP workforce, are all approaching retirement age, which will exacerbate the crisis in general practice.

Increased demand

The mismatch between available staff and health-service need is not just about supply problems; it is also about increasing demand. Not only are we supporting an ageing population, but there is no doubt that public expectation of the NHS has grown. The universal perception amongst staff is that activity has increased, and there are data supporting this impression. For example, between 1990 and 1998, emergency admissions to hospital rose by 28 per cent and overall acute hospital activity by 38 per cent (Buchan and Edwards 2000: 1067). Recent data produced by the Department of Health (DH 2003c) show that heart operations rose by 13 per cent in 2001–2 and a further 11 per cent in 2002–3, whilst there was an increase in first outpatient attendances from 8.5 million in 1987–8 to 13 million in 2002–3. Other areas of activity such as A&E attendances and radiological investigations have shown more modest increases.

Demand is not just a question of quantity; patients rightly expect care to be of a universally high quality and to be delivered in a timely fashion – and this cannot happen without adequately staffed services. In line with NHS targets, between October 2001 and September 2002 some 96 per cent of suspected cancer patients were seen by a specialist within two weeks of being urgently referred by their GP; this was an increase from 91 per cent the previous year. However, these numbers give little indication of quality of care, and such consultations are staff-intensive. Clinics for suspected cancer patients need to have sufficient doctors, nurses, therapists and support staff to communicate effectively with patients, to get their investigations completed, to give time for questions and to provide ongoing support and treatment. We saw in Chapter 2 how disastrous it was when an inexperienced junior doctor was left breaking bad news on his own.

Recruitment and retention issues

In addition to the problems in workforce-planning and increased demands on the service, the NHS is certainly not a monopoly employer. The public sector has always had to compete with the private sector for a large proportion of its workforce. One might anticipate many potential advantages of the private sector: better pay and working conditions, fewer staff shortages and a less stressful work environment. So why do over a million people choose to work in the NHS? The Audit Commission (2002) produced a detailed analysis of the motivators for recruitment and retention in the public sector. The top reasons for staff joining public services were 'to make a positive difference', 'to work with people/children', 'because it's what I always wanted to be' and 'to do interesting and rewarding work'. Interestingly, the public sector has a better track record for retaining staff than the private sector. Once employed, health-service employees express high satisfaction with their work (Pearson, Reilly and Robinson 2004). Important motivators are colleagues, training and development opportunities, and feeling valued and involved. Staff do not join the public sector for financial reward and, although lower pay has some impact on intention to leave, it ranks well below other factors such as being overwhelmed by bureaucracy, paperwork, targets, lack of autonomy and workload (Pearson, Reilly and Robinson 2004).

An important consideration for many staff groups is stress in the workplace. We have already touched on the stressors for GPs, but similar problems beset hospital staff and other sectors of the workforce. The proportion of doctors and other health professionals showing above-threshold levels of stress has stayed remarkably constant at around 28 per cent, compared with around 18 per cent in the general working population (Firth-Cozens 2003). Isobel Allen (2001) has studied stress factors in key hospital staff. For doctors, these include loss of autonomy, fear of making errors, increasing public expectations, isolation and loss of work–life balance. Senior nurses have different stressors, often focused around the staffing and resourcing of their wards, infrastructure problems, bed-management issues and externally imposed directives. In light of these pressures, it becomes a lot easier to understand why so many wards refused to give Peter Soames a bed, whether for Daniel or for the critically sick child who had fallen out of a treehouse and lay dying in Barnet.

For all staff groups, bullying in the workplace is a significant and worrying phenomenon. Bullying is, in part, a consequence of being under stress, and the 'caring professions' are not immune to this dysfunctional response. Sometimes the worst perpetrators are those in the most stressful work environments. But while this may be an explanation, it is not an excuse.

All these factors converge to make stress the commonest cause of sickness in NHS staff and a growing cause of concern for health-service policy-makers seeking ways to recruit and retain a healthy workforce with good morale.

Changes in professional training and working conditions

Because of the sheer numbers of nurses and doctors, relative to other clinical staff groups, major changes in the training of these two groups have had a knock-on effect on the workforce problems.

Prior to the 1990s, nursing and midwifery training was carried out in schools of nursing attached to the hospitals where students gained their clinical experience. Nursing and midwifery students were NHS employees, providing a direct contribution to patient care on hospital wards. In 1989, as part of a drive to improve the professional and academic base of nursing, Project 2000 was launched. Nurse-training was moved to a university setting as a degree or diploma subject, and student nurses ceased to be part of the staff establishment of each ward. They instead acquired a different status as trainees on ward placements. Their role was partially replaced by an increase in health-care assistants, but the loss of the service contribution, as well as the supervision requirements, put an additional workload on qualified nursing staff.

There have been two sets of changes to medical education, the first in 1996, aimed at the registrar grade, and a more recent set of changes initiated in 2004–5, aimed at the more junior grades of house officer and senior house officer. The combined effect has been to make training shorter and more structured. Doctors have always been well trained in technical skills, but there is now more emphasis on acquiring generic skills, such as communication, team-working and an understanding of ethics and governance – in fact all the areas emphasised as important within this book. Hopefully a doctor emerging from the new system will be better prepared for a consultation with the Johnsons than Sebastian was in Chapter 2.

Whilst improving the training culture, the changes have not been without their problems or their critics. Junior doctors (an unsatisfactory term used to describe any hospital doctor below consultant level) have now been rebadged as 'trainees'. This emphasises their need for supervision by consultant trainers. However, unlike student nurses, they are fully registered practitioners and are part of the hospital staff. Unsurprisingly, this gives a confusing and worrying message to patients, who expect to be treated by 'fully trained doctors'. With Project 2000 the nursing profession became more explicit about the service demarcation between students and trained staff, whilst the medical profession has become less so. There is thus considerable ambiguity about the role and service contribution of junior doctors, who are qualified professionals, are competent to undertake a large range of clinical tasks and are an important part of the workforce, and yet are labelled as 'trainees'.

To add to this climate of uncertainty, there has been a major employment change for junior doctors, and this has had a profound effect on the entire workforce. From August 2004, doctors in training have come under the auspices of the European Working Time Directive (EWTD), which puts tight constraints on the hours that they can work. The unacceptably long hours that junior doctors used to work – up to 100 hours a week – had already been considerably trimmed by previous legislation, but the EWTD regulations are more inflexible, are legally binding and carry severe penalties for NHS trusts if not rigorously implemented. The inescapable outcome is that there are not enough junior doctors to provide the same level of service and new solutions are being developed. Those solutions involve changing roles for other members of the health-care workforce.

Solutions: more staff, working differently

I tell you, sir, the only safeguard of order and discipline in the modern world is a standardized worker with interchangeable parts. That would solve the entire problem of management.
(Jean Giraudoux, French author and playwright [1882–1944])

The NHS Plan, with its promise of more investment and more NHS staff, was launched amidst considerable publicity in July 2000. A much quieter document preceded it – one that was not overtly in the public arena, but that contributed to many of the workforce considerations of the NHS Plan and its subsequent implementation. The report, *A Health Service of All the Talents: Developing the NHS Workforce* (Department of Health 2000a), acknowledged many of the workforce-planning and staffing problems outlined above, but it also made explicit the fact that remedying the situation was not just about adding staff. A far more radical change in education, culture and philosophy was needed to make the workforce more flexible and responsive. Tight professional hierarchies, boundaries and tribalism would need to be broken down in order to encourage a move to team-working.

Policy documents released since the publication of the NHS Plan have focused on both sides of this equation. More staff, working differently. Staff numbers are measurable, visible in the media and to the public, and hence politically high profile. An expansion of the workforce is dependent on either increasing the number of staff coming into the system or reducing the number leaving, and each of these aspects is being strongly tackled. But the success of the other side of the equation – the quieter, less visible revolution in driving new role development and replacing individual autonomy with team-working – will ultimately be just as important to the success of the NHS.

It is beyond the scope of this book to discuss all aspects of this in detail. In this section we will focus on a few issues that are of philosophical or practical importance and that are relevant to Daniel's story.

Further information on good human-resources practice within the NHS can be found on the Department of Health web site.

Attracting and retaining more staff

More money does not automatically buy more staff. There is a long 'lag phase' because of the time taken to train new clinicians. Increasing consultant numbers from internal growth is a particular challenge, because of the very long interval from medical student to consultant: a minimum of fourteen years under the current system and longer in some of the skill-based specialities such as surgery. Hence, there is a tension between the medical profession and the Government about proposals to shorten the training time, with doctors remaining anxious about a fall in standards.

Strategies to increase staff recruitment and retention have therefore had to be multi-modal, and the key strands are:

- improving retention by making the NHS a better place to work;
- increasing training places for professional staff;
- active 'return to work policies' for those who have left the service;
- international recruitment.

Strategies aimed at improving retention (which fall under the banner Improving Working Lives) are broad ranging and include more flexible and child-friendly working arrangements, encouraging staff diversity, providing learning and development opportunities and various pay-structure changes (Agenda for Change, Consultant Contract, GP Contract). An important plank is to reduce bullying in the workplace, which has already been highlighted as a worrying issue. Elimination of bullying requires strong leadership and a zero-tolerance approach from the top of the organisation.

Hopefully some of you who are reading this book are interested because you are considering a career in the NHS. The NHS Careers web site <http://www.nhscareers.nhs.uk/> or telephone service (0845 60 60 655) are helpful sources of information. For those considering returning to work in the NHS, the following may be helpful:

Box 4.1 Learning points for potential staff: returning to work in the NHS

- What you need to do in order to return to professional practice depends on how long you have been away, what you have been doing outside of the NHS and what professional qualifications you have.
- New practice requirements mean that nurses, midwives and health visitors who return after a gap will usually have to complete a return-to-nursing, midwifery or health-visiting course before starting a job. For other professional groups the situation is variable. However, you are under a professional obligation to be a competent practitioner and this is likely to involve you undertaking some preparatory refresher work. Those planning to return to a NHS profession should contact their professional body directly in order to find out about returning requirements.
- Financial support may be available to help those required to undertake return-to-practice training and NHS trusts, strategic health authorities and workforce development confederations can be contacted for further information.
- Age is no barrier to returning. What's important is your motivation.
- Flexible working opportunities are excellent within the NHS and information about what is offered locally can be gained by contacting the relevant trust's personnel department.
- NHS Careers (0845 60 60 655) can offer information on returning to practice in the NHS and will give you details of the local return to practice coordinator.

With international recruitment still an essential part of the strategy, questions have to be asked about the ethics of this practice. James Buchan (2004: 10) discusses a number of different dimensions surrounding this controversial issue, focusing particularly on the need for both ethical recruitment (that is, not stripping developing countries of professional staff) and ethical employment (that is, equitable treatment of overseas staff). He also notes the importance of not oversimplifying; there are push factors from the provider countries, such as lack of career prospects and threat of violence, as well as pull factors from the UK and others.

Since 1999 there have been guidelines on which countries it is ethically acceptable for the NHS to recruit from, and these were revamped in 2001. In 2004, the Department of Health announced an intention to tighten up on these guidelines to reduce 'back-door' recruitment to the NHS after initial entry through the private sector, which operates outside the NHS guidelines. It is a fine line, and one which will need constant vigilance, as indicated by John Hutton when he launched the new guidelines:

> We are determined not to destabilise the health-care system of developing countries. The NHS is expanding, but we're not going to do that at the expense of other countries.
> (John Hutton, Department of Health Press Release,
> August 2004)

Working differently

Users of the NHS will have encountered staff from all backgrounds taking on a variety of new roles. For example, a physiotherapy team in Kent provides home support to patients with respiratory problems so they can mange their condition without coming into hospital every time. In North Bristol a community-liaison pharmacist is responsible for the discharge of complex patients, and community pharmacists are taking a more active role in giving front-line public health advice on stopping smoking and sexual health, as well as running some specific pharmacist-led clinics. Nurses are taking on a variety of new roles, including surgical admission clinics, primary-care assessment clinics, and so on.

In all these examples, novel and different use of staff is helping to address some of the shortfalls arising from recruitment problems and the EWTD for doctors. However, that alone is not an adequate reason for putting new roles in place: unless these changes can be shown to provide better, more accessible and safer care for patients, as well as a sensible career structure for those undertaking them, they cannot be justified. New roles should not be introduced merely to put sticking plaster on the cracks in the NHS – they must be about improved services.

There is nothing extraordinary about the notion that staff should be undertaking new roles; it would be more worrying to find staff continuing to work in exactly the same way that they were ten or twenty years ago. We no longer incarcerate patients for months in tuberculosis sanatoria. Clinical medicine has changed dramatically – first, in reducing the need for extended hospital admissions and in providing more community-based care, and, second, in using technologies that were not even conceived of a few years ago.

The rest cure, Firland Tuberculosis Sanatorium (1911–43)

Firland nurses were expected to train patients in the Way of the Cure with missionary zeal, to model and enforce discipline, and to maintain a spotlessly hygienic environment. Any thoughts or activities that 'heated the blood' were forbidden. Director Stith assigned older, more mature nurses to care for the men, in the hope that the men's libidos would remain at rest. Non-sexual activities considered harmful included 'letter writing, reading, and letting the mind dwell on any subject which hurries the circulation'.

(Becker 2002)

There are many examples of how changed roles have benefited patients. This is not surprising since the traditional allocation of tasks and roles between different professional groups has, in part, been an arbitrary development, and not necessarily based on the best person for the job. There is already evidence accumulating that nurses are as good or better than doctors at managing routine surgical admissions (Jones et al. 2000: 261), while a detailed review of the literature shows that patients are more satisfied with nurse practitioners than doctors as a first point of contact in primary care, with no difference in health outcomes (Horrocks et al. 2002: 819).

Nonetheless, new solutions breed new questions and dilemmas. The nursing profession faces a complex issue: nurses are rightly developing advanced skills in specialist areas and leading a range of services, and yet there is also a strong need to retain basic nursing skills. However specialist the paediatric ward, the nursing staff should still be able to manage Daniel's portacath. Susan Lowson, nurse adviser to the Health Service Ombudsman, reports that what patients want most from a nurse is to spend time with them, and that complaints about

nurses were most commonly about a failure to deliver the basics
(Parish 2004: 14). Defining and maintaining the unique contribution
of nursing, whilst also developing highly specialist practitioners, is a
difficult juggling act and is set to become even more difficult as new
role development continues to offer not only new opportunities and
challenges, but also new pressures on the balance between breadth
and depth of knowledge and skills.

> We need an image of nurses who are knowledgeable and skilled,
> yet also caring and compassionate. Accepting the notion of an
> integrated art and science of professional practice. Nurses who
> develop new skills and knowledge for the benefit of patients but
> never lose sight of the fundamental values of human caring that
> define and inform professional practice.
>
> (Mullally 2003)

Box 4.2 Learning points for staff: reflecting on roles

- Is a given patient's condition or needs so unusual that most staff could not care for them?
- Has increasing specialisation led to staff being unfamiliar with more general needs?
- Is it time to rethink ways of working to ensure that care can be provided for patients who may be placed on any ward?
- Reflect on your own care provision and that of the ward team. Do these always meet the standards you would expect to receive yourself or to be provided for your relatives?
- Ask yourself whether you could provide better care by doing something differently or by working more efficiently with others or across teams.

THE SOCIETAL CONTEXT: TIERS, TEAMS AND TRIBALISM

> Oh Great Spirit, keep me from ever judging a man until I've walked a mile in his moccasins.
>
> (Sioux Indian Prayer)

The barriers to new ways of working are not just about the tension between acquiring new skills and maintaining old ones. They are not even about public acceptance of new roles; patients generally make rapid and accurate judgements about the experience and competence of a practitioner and are less concerned about their professional background. To understand one of the major barriers, we have to go back to a third-grade classroom in Iowa in 1968, the day after Martin Luther King was shot dead in Memphis.

Jane Elliot, a third-grade teacher in an all-white, all-Christian community launched a brave and dangerous experiment, later know as 'Blue-Eyed/Brown-Eyed'. Appalled at the assassination and at a loss to explain racism and discrimination to her students, she was reminded of the Sioux prayer above. She concluded that the only way to make her children understand was to make them 'walk in another man's moccasins'. So she divided the class on the basis of eye colour and began praising those with brown eyes, telling them how gifted and talented they were, and ridiculing, demeaning and marginalising those with blue eyes. Within a few short hours, she had generated an in-group and an out-group and had produced an extraordinary level of prejudicial behaviour between the two groups of children that divided friendships and erupted into playground violence by the first recess. The next day, she reversed the process, making the underdogs into the dominant group.

The experiment gained national and international fame and has been widely used in equal-opportunities training. The focus was initially on racial discrimination and, as such, seems rather removed from discussions about new roles. In fact, Jane Elliot's experiment is an example of very basic human behaviours: tribalism and ethnocentrism. A tribe is any group of people that perceives itself as distinct, and that is so perceived by the outside world. The group might be a race, but it need not be; it can just as well be a religious sect, a political group or an occupational group (Van der Dennen 1985). Tribes go on to behave in an ethnocentric manner; they treat their 'in-group' members with loyalty, cohesion and solidarity, and they develop a shared value-set and a belief in the superiority of the group. There is a powerful human drive to 'belong', and the bigger and more powerful the group we belong to, the more secure we feel. By definition, the 'out-group' is perceived as inferior, and various negative constructs are applied to its members. Racism and xenophobia are extreme examples, but far more minor examples occur on a day-to-day basis in every walk of life. For example, those who are not computer literate will stereotype 'computer techies' as nerds; we admire the acting elite, while branding them as 'lovies' and deriding their magazine-cover lifestyle; and those who are not blessed with sporting prowess may apply a 'knucklehead' image to those who spend their time working out. Even outside of Hogwarts Academy children are divided into 'houses' at school and, in later life, into teams at work. They are part of a nation or a club or a firm.

It is important to understand, therefore, that ethnocentrism is part of the human condition. We all use social identity to draw in-group/out-group boundaries. Whilst ethnocentrism can lead to malign behaviours, people can, of course, be socialised to be proud of their identity or heritage without necessarily hating or demeaning others. The trick is to engender the pride without encouraging the hatred.

Professional ethnocentrism

Professional ethnocentrism is alive and well and living in the NHS (Nyatanga 1998). A special combined issue of the *BMJ* and *Nursing Times*, published in April 2000, explored some of the problems. While the focus was on doctors and nurses, the issues translate much more broadly to interprofessional divisions across the Health Service; divisions that can interfere with team work and new-role development.

The game that is played out between doctors and nurses is rehearsed from the earliest playground enactments right up to the senior tiers of the two professions. It has been reflected in countless *Carry On* films and James Robertson Justice stereotypes. The previous generation's Dr Kildare and Dr Finlay have been supplanted by George Clooney's far more heart-stopping Dr Doug Ross of *ER*. The image is emblazoned in many miles of celluloid. Doctors are portrayed as gods; they have the authority, the status, the power to cure, and the social and financial rewards that follow, while nurses are angels of mercy, handmaidens to the gods, and the guardians of holistic care and the patient perspective.

An article by Celia Davies (2000) stands out in providing a more mature exploration of the realities that underlie and generate these stereotypes. Medical training has traditionally focused on developing doctors who are self-reliant and independent. Expertise, autonomy and responsibility have been valued over interdependence, deliberation and dialogue, and the expectations of patients and colleagues have reinforced this value set. Nurses have responded by 'working around' doctors, accepting a subservient role and making behind-the-scenes suggestions that allow the doctor to maintain apparent control over the decision-making process. Both professions need to change their culture and behaviour if the new roles that are being established are to be successful.

The traditional medical model is already in the process of deconstruction with the increasing focus on patient choice and partnership, which will be explored in more detail in later chapters. The increasingly academic base that has been developed in nursing through Project 2000 and its downstream changes, and the increasing focus on generic-skills training in medicine outlined earlier in this chapter might be expected to facilitate a recasting of the relationship between doctors and nurses. However, to some extent, the new role development that has occurred because of restrictions in junior doctors' hours and the shortfall in medical time may have a detrimental effect if not correctly understood and interpreted. This is because it has shifted the focus from the development of the nursing profession in its own right to nurses' ability to 'substitute' for medical roles. Evaluation, including some of the references cited earlier in this chapter, is at an unsophisticated stage, and is based on whether nurses can do tasks as well as or better than doctors. But the strength of teams lies not in substitution, but in difference. A case study from Great Ormond Street will be used to highlight this point.

The sum is greater than the parts

Great Ormond Street was the first hospital in the country to launch a special team to look after the hospital overnight, replacing a large number of doctors all working in isolation with a dedicated team comprising three paediatricians and two intensive-care-trained nurses (known as Clinical Site Practitioners or CSPs) (Cass et al. 2003: 270). One of the CSPs leads the team each night, chairs a formal handover from the day staff and assigns work in an organised way. The team then meets up again to review the sickest patients and take a break together.

Resistance to the plan was substantial. Staff were afraid that this small team would not have enough people or the expertise to look after the hospital safely. In addition, the reversal of the normal hierarchy, with a nurse managing the doctors, was professional heresy.

A huge number of lessons were learnt in the early days of the team. The most immediate lesson was that the carefully structured team was better able to manage the workload, including emergencies, largely because the team model was simply more efficient than the previous model of doctors working in isolation. But the most important lesson was that patient care was better, because the team was able to share expertise and responsibility in decision-making and to learn from each other's skills and knowledge. The CSPs had the best-developed skills for assessing critically ill children, whilst the doctors were skilled in diagnosis and treatment. The two components were brought together in a partnership.

There were teething problems. For example, the fact that the CSPs could take blood and put in drips meant that some of the doctors expected that they would always be there to do this for them. But it wasn't always appropriate for the CSP, as the most senior and experienced clinician on site, to be doing this when they might be needed for something that required their unique skill set. However, things quickly settled down as members of the team came to understand that they each had unique skills to bring to the party, and when it came to equally shared skill sets, it was down to the least busy person at the time.

Doctors are, of course, used to working in teams, but the traditional structure has been hierarchical and consultant focused, with each consultant having his or her 'firm' of juniors. The shift-working imposed by shorter hours for junior doctors has put an end to this pattern and the new teams are multi-professional. This requires a greater degree of inter-professional as well as intra-professional trust and interdependence, characteristics that, as described previously, are novel to the medical culture, but which are gaining ground at a growing pace.

We are starting to see evidence that team-working improves care for patients (Baggs et al. 1999: 1991). Having a team-based approach can help with a huge range of tasks and can ensure optimum use of beds for the many Daniels who need them. For example, various appropriately constituted multi-professional teams can take over the management of severe pain relief across a hospital, can give nutritional and feeding advice or plan hospital discharge – all of which can make inpatient care more efficient and effective and can help patients to get home faster and more safely. There are also lessons to be learnt from aeronautical settings, which demonstrate that less hierarchical teams are safer because they allow freer communication (Firth-Cozens 2001: ii26). Teams may still need leaders, but they need a different style of leader compared with more traditional single-profession groups.

Teams need to learn together in order to maximise the benefit of group experience. However, the initial professional education socialises nursing students to be nurses and medical students to be doctors, often at the expense of inter-professional team working or identity (Nyatanga and Forman 2002). We do not yet have good evidence as to whether those clinicians who experienced interprofessional learning as students are any less likely to fall prey to professional ethnocentrism or to fare better in the new models of care. Meanwhile, we have to consider how to foster good joint learning and team-working amongst the greater majority of the current workforce, which has came through traditional mono-professional education routes. Nyatanga and Forman (2002) suggest that we need to recategorise or reframe the in-group/out-group boundaries, so that the in-group is redefined at a more inclusive level as the team within which professionals work. This approach is not without its pitfalls. Established professional boundaries are hard to change. Nonetheless the GOSH night team has melded well and transcends the professional boundaries of its constituent members.

The drive to tribalism is strong and will continue to present challenges, wherever the boundaries are drawn. Nonetheless, it is timely to lay to rest some of the more unproductive stereotypes which have hampered true inter-professional working over an extended period.

AT THE FRONT LINE: MAKING A DIFFERENCE

Professor David Baum, the first president of the College of Paediatrics and Child Health, was an international pioneer, promoting children's well-being across the world. Sadly, he died of a heart attack whilst on a sponsored cycle ride to raise money for child health services in Kosovo and Gaza. He was fond of telling the following parable, which has become the symbol of his appeal fund:

The parable of the starfish

An old man walking on the beach at dawn noticed a boy picking up a starfish and throwing it into the sea. When asked why, the boy explained that the stranded starfish would die if left to lie in the morning sun. 'But there are millions of starfish on this beach,' said the old man. 'How can your efforts make a difference?' The boy picked up another starfish and placed it in the waves. 'It makes a difference to this one,' he said.

(In memoriam, David Baum [1940–99])

The themes highlighted in this chapter sound huge and intractable. It would be easy for anyone at the front line to feel overwhelmed by the demands, the targets, the staffing shortages, the inspections, the conflicting priorities – to feel that there is nothing they can do to make a difference. And yet staff can and do make a difference on a daily basis, not only to individual patients but also by coming up with innovative solutions to practical problems at the coal face.

When the Snakes and Ladders drama was staged at GOSH, the 'No room at the inn' episode was the most controversial, because it challenged everyone: the efficiency of the cleaners, the bed-blocking practices of the doctors, the over-specialisation of the nurses, the organisational skills of the managers.

Why did this particular episode make everyone in the audience feel so uncomfortable? Probably because they knew that everyone in the drama had a choice. Susan chose not to accept that there was no bed for Daniel and found her way through to the bed manager. Peter didn't throw away the yellow sticky with Daniel's name on it as soon as he put the phone down on Susan, nor did he pass the problem on to someone else. Instead he decided to make an effort to get him admitted. The staff nurse on Barry Ward chose not to get someone to show her how to use a portacath; instead she refused Daniel's admission. The sister on Prior had spent months taking the path of least resistance and not challenging the consultant who persistently blocked beds on her ward. And Millie on Davenport Ward decided that she had too much going on to call domestic services for the third time that morning about the cubicle that needed cleaning. But then, she thought again, and she made the extra effort. Everyone made their personal choices about whether they could make a difference to 'one more starfish'. Peter made one more choice. He decided to apologise to Millie for snapping at her on the phone.

Personal responsibility and organisational culture

The reality is that however hard we try, some problems can't be fixed. Peter might have been able to find a bed that day for Daniel, or he might not. As it happened, he did. However, one piece of 'local knowledge' that everyone acquires after working for a short time in an organisation – whether in the NHS or not – is who to phone with a problem. We can distinguish the 'can-do' from the 'can't-do' colleagues.

At GOSH, the Chief Executive has launched a Personal Responsibility Framework aimed at encouraging staff to take more active responsibility for all facets of their daily work lives – and on the flip side, to reduce bullying and negative and dysfunctional behaviours. The information given earlier in this chapter about what attracts people into the NHS highlights the fact that for the most part, it is dependent on the goodwill of a workforce which is there because its members want to make a difference. They are, to a large degree, predisposed to 'can-do' behaviours. Equally clearly, they also sometimes feel worn down by the bureaucracy, the paperwork and the unrealistic demands – and colleagues bullying or harassing them can be the last straw. In Peter's case, his response to Millie was probably an understandable one-off irritation from someone under pressure, and an action he regretted immediately. For some staff, these behaviours are more persistent.

Why should sensible, considerate and responsible behaviour need writing into a Personal Responsibility Framework? Surely this is so self-evident, it does not need to be said? The answer is 'yes and no'; 'yes' because we do all know it, and 'no' because none of us can claim to consistently do it. So writing it down and agreeing a value-set is a way of developing an organisational culture in which taking responsibility is valued and bullying is seen as a negative, rather than a 'macho' behaviour.

To service users and, perhaps, to staff, it may seem a little odd to talk about organisations having a 'culture'. But although it is not a concept that people are immediately aware of, once the idea is floated, most people can immediately relate to it. For example, in the United Kingdom, Marks & Spencer has developed an image as a 'good employer'. More broadly, without even visiting Harvard or Silicon Valley, many people would have an image of the culture they might encounter in a formal American academic institution compared to a computer corporation.

As soon as we understand the concept, it raises all sorts of questions. What creates an organisational culture, and how is it changed and developed? How can there be 'an organisational culture' when an organisation consists of a huge mix of different individuals? Is organisational culture important? And is it the same in all NHS hospitals, given that they work to the same philosophies and principles?

A useful definition of organisational culture is 'the unique configuration of norms, values, beliefs, ways of behaving and so on, that characterize the manner in which groups and individuals combine to get things done', and Iles and Sutherland (2001: 32–3) have discussed the importance of different kinds of organisational cultures in managing change in health-care settings. In other words, organisations are coalitions of individuals, and organisational culture is the glue that holds them together and that gives the organisation a sense of commitment and identity (see Bolman and Deal 1997 for a more detailed analysis of these issues). In general, those who identify with the organisational beliefs, ethos and value-set will stay, and those who do not will leave, so the culture becomes self-perpetuating. This means that culture is important not just for retaining staff, but also for determining how the organisation makes decisions and how its core values are maintained.

It is unrealistic to expect everyone to be on top form every day, to always go the extra mile and never to be irritable with colleagues or patients. The NHS is staffed by real people, who have rows with their boyfriends and girlfriends, have financial worries, get drenched in the rain on the way to work, and are sometimes feeling unwell themselves. But if everyone went the extra mile just one more time each week, whether in their dealings with patients or colleagues, that would make a difference to more than a million starfish.

Box 4.3 Learning points for staff: dealing with inappropriate behaviours and bullying in the workplace

- If you think someone is behaving inappropriately, try speaking to the person directly. In most trusts you can get help on how to do this from the trust's Harassment and Bullying Guidance.

continued

- If you don't feel able to do this, you can get support and advice from your manager, your manager's manager or another senior person in your department.
- Many training departments offer training in assertion skills, communication skills and how to deal with conflict. If they do not have in-house courses, they will be able to advise you on where you can get this training.

Other people who you can approach are:

- A representative from your union or professional body.
- The trust's counselling service.
- Your personnel officer.

The following are useful contact numbers:

- RCN Direct on 0845 772 6100 (for RCN members).
- BMA Helpline on 0845 920 0169 (for BMA members).
- Unison Direct on 0845 355 0845 (for Unison members).
- Andrea Adams Helpline on 01273 704 900 (for all staff).

Box 4.4 Learning points for staff: dealing with work-related stress

Inappropriate behaviour sometimes happens when people are under stress. Many trusts offer counselling services, which are an excellent source of free and confidential help for a wide range of personal and work-related problems. In addition to the helplines given above, the following agencies can help with particular problems:

- Drinkline: open to people with alcohol problems, their families, friends, carers and colleagues on 0800 917 8282 in confidence.
- National Drugs Helpline: open to people with drug-misuse problems, their families, friends, carers and colleagues on 0800 776 600.

Getting involved

Sometimes, an overwhelming frustration for both patients and staff is the feeling that things are just not being done in the most sensible or effective way. The mother sitting at the bedside of her child for weeks or the husband sitting at the bedside of his wife might be in a position to spot inefficiencies or duplication of effort that are not obvious to the staff who have been doing things that way for several years. Equally, it could be the most junior physiotherapist or the new ward pharmacist who stumbles upon a time-consuming or convoluted procedure, but feels powerless to speak up about it.

A measure of the leadership and openness of the ward or department is the ability to respond to and incorporate suggestions from patients, newcomers and junior staff. There are, of course, ways and ways of planting new ideas. On a day that two staff are off sick and an unbooked patient has just arrived, it is probably not a good idea to approach the ward sister with an observation such as 'It's amazing that you have such an archaic system for organising patients' drugs for discharge here. We had a similar system where I used to work, but it was ditched over five years ago.' The next box offers suggestions for approaches that are more likely to be successful:

Box 4.5 Learning points for staff: getting involved in changing a local process

Option 1: Choose your moment and just say it. If you have spotted a system or process that you would like to see changed, then try picking a quiet, non-stressful moment to say something. The ward team may well be delighted with your suggestion.

Option 2: If you think there will be resistance, take a more subtle approach:

- Have a chat to a colleague and see if anyone else has suggested that change is necessary.
- Pick an opportune moment to have a chat to your manager or the ward sister, as appropriate. Highlight the problems you have noticed and ask about why things are done in this way. There may be a good reason. There may not be a good reason!

---

continued

- Suggest your alternative and see if they are receptive to the possibility.

Option 3: Inviting involvement from others:

- Approach your manager or ward sister and ask if you could get involved in an audit or evaluation of the process as part of your own personal development.
- Working with other people on the audit is a good way to get involved in a team project and to learn about how to gather and make sense of information.
- Once you have gathered data on current performance, the results may well speak for themselves about the need for change.
- Ask if you can feed back the results at a ward or team meeting. This will involve everyone in thinking about the problem and possible solutions.

Option 4: Joining an existing process review team:

- In many wards and departments, there will be a team working on a number of projects to change processes and to make them more patient-focused.
- Volunteer to join the team. Even if the team is not looking for new members, you may be able to sit in as an observer on a couple of occasions.
- Try channelling your idea through someone who is an established member of the team.
- Joining such a team is a good way of learning about change processes, even if you don't come in with an idea of your own.

Many processes go beyond an individual ward or department. Some of the thorniest problems involve issues that cut across the organisation. Take the consultant who was guilty of 'bed-blocking'. What made him behave that way? The probable answer was that he was under pressure himself to meet targets on his waiting list for admission, and if his own ward was filled with 'outliers' (patients like Daniel, under the care of other teams), then he could not admit his own patients. That would have an impact on the income and activity figures of his particular department. How should this consultant balance the need to do his best for his own patients with the need to be sensitive to the requirements of the rest of the hospital? We need guidelines on managing beds and waiting lists that encompass the whole hospital: after this particular episode of Snakes and Ladders a number of staff volunteered to try to help draw up such a set of guidelines for GOSH.

Box 4.6 Learning points for staff: getting involved in organisational change

- If you are a little more senior and are interested in getting involved in change outside your immediate ward area, discuss this with your manager.
- Managers are frequently involved in many trust-level committees, and are often very ready to bring new blood on board.

Another important personal responsibility is not only to stay up to date with current developments, but also to make sure that you do not lose your broad-based professional skills. One important role of the CSP team described earlier in the chapter is to provide support to ward teams so they feel able to look after patients with less familiar problems or illnesses that require a different skill set to the patients who are more usually on the ward.

Box 4.7 Learning points for staff: personal development

- Every member of staff should have regular appraisals and should have a Personal Development Plan (PDP). This will be all the more important with the advent of Agenda for Change, the major pay-review system for NHS staff.
- In thinking about your personal development, remember the need to maintain breadth as well as depth and to include relevant generic skills training in your plans.

---

continued

- If you think you might like to undertake a new role, your appraisal will be an ideal time to discuss this with your manager, and to get the training built into your PDP. If you don't have an imminent appraisal, but have a good idea about how you could extend your role, flag it up with your manager at a suitable one-to-one meeting.
- Your trust training department may be a good resource to find out about training opportunities and funding that might help you in developing new skills.
- The Department of Health web site has a database listing new-role developments for many different staff. If you'd like to be doing something different, but are not sure what, it is worth visiting the site.

As a patient, this is an ideal time to get involved. Public policy is firmly directed towards user involvement in planning and improving services. There is a clear move away from the NHS staff acting as 'expert advisers' to a partnership model of working. There are both formal and informal ways to get involved, and some examples are as follows:

Table 4.1 Expert adviser versus partnership model

Expert adviser	Partnership
Define patient needs	Elicit patient needs
Give advice	Discuss options
Solve problems	Explore solutions
Decide what information they need	Ask what information they want
Encourage dependency	Empower and enable

Source: *Improvement Leaders' Guide to Involving Parents and Carers*, Modernisation Agency. Crown copyright material is reproduced with the permission of the Controller of HMSO and the Queen's Printer for Scotland.

Box 4.8 Learning points for patients: getting involved (informal mechanisms)

- If you have been an inpatient or a carer of an inpatient on a ward, and have some ideas about change, approach the ward sister and ask if the team needs a patient representative on any of their improvement-planning groups.
- If you are going to join a group, remember to check up on the practicalities: How often will it meet? At what time of the day? And how will your expenses be reimbursed?
- If they do not have a regular planning group, they may well want patients who will respond to questionnaires about the service and about how to improve it, or to come to one or two targeted meetings about issues on which they have expertise.
- If you have ideas about how things could be changed – either at ward level or more broadly in the hospital, but feel that you are not being taken seriously by the ward staff, go and talk to the PALS adviser for the hospital (see Chapter 2).
- If you have expertise in a particular condition or would be prepared to give support and advice to other patients and families, let the ward staff know; it is always helpful to have contact families for those who are coming to terms with new diagnoses or problems.
- Sometimes patients are the best teachers, and many courses value having patients or carers to talk to medical students, trainee nurses or therapists about their condition. It is always helpful to have contact details for patients who would be prepared to do this.

Box 4.9 Learning points for patients: getting involved (formal mechanisms)

- Patient and Public Involvement Forums are more formal bodies that have been set up for every PCT and NHS trust.
- Their role is to obtain views from local communities, to make recommendations about how the service should be

continued

delivered and to influence the design and access to NHS services.

- The time commitment is about two to three hours per week, and members do not have to have particular start-up skills, but will be given any training that they need after joining.
- Further information and application forms can be downloaded from the Commission for Patient and Public Involvement in Health web site <http://www.cppih.org>.

Box 4.10 Learning points for staff: dealing with resource pressures

- The NHS Plan sets out a new relationship with patients and families: treatment and care must be shaped around their needs and lives, not vice versa.
- Always keep in mind the distress caused by waiting for treatment especially when in pain or seriously ill. Consider the effect on families: disrupted home life, stress, and so on, when admissions don't go as planned.
- Always include a length-of-stay estimate when planning admissions to allow more efficient bed use.
- Letters to patients or families about admission should include a paragraph about the risk of cancellation or the bed not being available at the planned time.
- Ask families what they think about the care you provide and to tell you honestly what they find helpful or what falls short of their expectations. Do not rely on complaints to tell you if there are problems or assume that silence implies satisfaction.

At the end of the day

Peter hadn't been so relieved to see the end of a shift in months. He decided he couldn't quite face the Tube yet so, on an impulse, he decided to pop up to Davenport, apologise to Millie in person and to see if the Johnson boy's admission had gone OK. When he reached the ward, Millie had her coat on and was just heading out of the door with Jane, the service manager and a man Peter hadn't met before.

'Hi Peter,' Millie said, as they converged at the ward entrance. 'What brings you up to Davenport at this time of the evening?'

Peter instantly felt rather embarrassed to be caught on the hop like this, particularly in front of Jane and a complete stranger. But on the spur of the moment, he couldn't come up with anything other than the truth. 'Well, actually I came by to thank you for taking the Johnson boy for me, and to apologise for being so short-tempered earlier on.'

'Oh, don't be daft. I didn't think anything of it,' Millie replied instantly. 'We're just about to go to the George for a quick drink. Want to come?'

Peter was delighted to accept. He discovered en route to the pub that the other man was Jane's husband Yiannos, and that he was a banker in the City.

'Good God, what a terrible day,' Peter said, when they had settled into a smoky corner of the pub and he'd taken a first long pull from his pint. 'It went from bad to worse after I spoke to you, Millie. Every possible bed crisis you can imagine, short of a busload of children crashing outside the hospital. I spent two hours this afternoon trying to find a bed for a child for spinal surgery. There'd been a muddle because the ward thought he'd cancelled with a cold, so they gave the bed to another child . . . and then he turned up anyway.'

'So why didn't they just send him home?' Yiannos asked.

'Well, as the parents were sure that they hadn't rung in to cancel, it would have been classed as a hospital cancellation . . . and apparently we're sailing close to the wind on cancelled operations, so the Surgical General Manager was in a complete twitch because she reckoned it might tip the balance on our star rating, and drop us from three to two.'

Yiannos looked at Peter in disbelief. 'Do you mean to tell me that one cancellation of one boy's surgery could make difference to your star rating?'

'Well, probably not,' Peter admitted. 'But if there's an arbitrary line somewhere, and we're running close to it, I guess it doesn't take much to push us one way or the other. The trouble is that targets just end up making people feel on edge all the time about things like this.'

'That's right,' said Jane. 'I'm glad I'm on the medical side, because so many more of the targets are surgical. One of the surgery service managers has been off sick for weeks, and I'm sure it's stress-related.'

'But these star ratings . . . do they show how good the care is?' Yiannos asked.

'Not really,' Jane said. 'It's more about stuff you can count or measure, like trolley waits in casualty and how good patients think the food is. There are a few crude indicators of how good surgeons are . . . like how many patients die after bypass surgery. But a lot of the stuff we do in paediatrics just isn't measurable in that way. Anyway, I gather the whole star-rating system is going to be scrapped next year, and replaced with something else.'

'Just as well,' Peter said. 'When I was at Fettsham, the hospital went down to a zero-star rating. One of my neighbours, whose son was under Fettsham for his epilepsy got really worried about it and came and asked me if she should get him transferred somewhere else. I told her no way. The children's department there was fantastic. The hospital's rating had only dropped because of overspending, and that had nothing to do with how good the care was. But you can see what it does to public confidence.'

'You probably haven't heard then,' said Jane. 'I gather they're trying to close most of the acute services at Fettsham, and move them all over to Hannam General.'

'No, I hadn't heard.' Peter was clearly upset. 'I haven't been in touch with anyone there since we moved down to London. Has the local press got hold of it yet?'

'No, I happened to hear because my cousin works in Accounts there, and they're all pretty gutted about it. Usual story. Not a big enough critical mass of medical staff to make the acute on-call rotas safe since the working-time directive. And with the nursing shortages as well, they can't run specialist services on both sites. It's Kidderminster revisited.'

'Kidderminster? What happened there then?' Yiannos asked.

'Similar scenario,' Jane said. 'Kidderminster was one of three hospitals in Worcestershire, all serving a relatively small population. Kidderminster was definitely the weakest link. It was the smallest, it had no paediatric department because training recognition had been withdrawn, there was only one A&E consultant and four surgeons. And they were about to lose recognition from the College of Surgeons because they were too small to train junior doctors. Plus, to make matters worse, the Health Authority had a 20 million pound deficit. So the big idea was to merge all the services on a new hospital site in Worcester and, hey presto, clinical and financial problems solved in one hit.'

'Sounds fine to me,' Yiannos said. 'As a banker, I have to say this sounds like the first sensible idea I've heard out of the NHS all evening.'

'Well, you might not have thought that if you lived in Kidderminster. At least, the local people certainly didn't. They launched a strong media campaign, with a raft of stories about how many people would die in ambulances on the way to Worcester. The fact is that people had probably died already at Kidderminster because of poor quality care, but that did not come to light in the coverage.

'Anyway, they looked to David Lock, their local MP, for support. He was swayed by the clinical data – so he said that he couldn't support the local campaigners because he thought the Health Authority proposals were right. So then suddenly a retired Kidderminster consultant appeared, took up the local cause, and stood for election against Lock. Result – Lock lost a completely safe Labour seat at the next election, and ever since then the Government has been terrified of the words "reconfiguration of health services".'

'Well there's bound to be an election in the next six months,' Yiannos said. 'So it looks like Fettsham is pretty secure in the immediate future. Another round, anyone?'

UNRESOLVED QUESTIONS: INFORMED CHOICE

> The public are uninformed purchasers of health care.
>
> (Lock 2002)

The David Lock story is real. Few can doubt David Lock's integrity or his belief that he was doing the right thing in not supporting the local population in their campaign to keep Kidderminster Hospital open. No one commits political suicide lightly. Some might criticise his actions on the basis that he was elected to represent the views of his constituents, even if that duty was at odds with his conscience. But his comment above, made during the course of a presentation to the Royal College of Paediatrics and Child Health in 2002, is an important one. It did not reflect disappointment in the constituents who failed to re-elect him, but rather in the failure of the Health Authority and those supporting the change to communicate effectively with the public and to provide them with accessible and timely information. He went on to make the point that the Health Authority does not 'own' the NHS; it is 'owned' by the public who use it and pay for it. In Kidderminster, they made their decision on the basis of locality, loyalty and external appearances. Had they been given better information about clinical outcomes, they might have made a different decision. On the other hand, plummeting confidence in national- and local-government data might have compromised trust in the information.

By launching formally constituted Patient and Public Involvement Forums, the Government has shown a clear intent to involve users in making choices, not just about their own treatment, but about a range of planning and delivery issues for their local services. This is not a new idea; a commission involving both professional and lay members was set up to decide how to ration health care in Oregon as long ago as the early 1990s (Klein 1991: 1). Support and training for forum members will ensure that these bodies go well beyond tokenism and serve an important local function. However, many more people need to understand the issues as they choose to 'vote' in a variety of ways – through campaigns such as that at Kidderminster, through responding to public consultations and, ultimately, at the ballot box.

Dilemmas and good practice in informing patients about their own treatment options are covered in detail in later chapters. This is territory that is familiar for health-care providers. They are less used to presenting information about the broader complexities of health-care provision so that the public can make truly informed choices. So what kind of information is needed, and how should it be presented?

Lessons were learnt from Kidderminster, and the Department of Health (2003b) launched guidelines on how to redesign services in a more collaborative way. Nonetheless, the current administration has placed a growing emphasis on targets and performance indicators. If the Government is to demonstrate progress in achieving the promises made in the NHS Plan and subsequent documents, it must have quantifiable data. Similarly, if patients are to be encouraged to make choices between Hospital A and Hospital B for their treatment, they need data to inform that choice.

In July 2004, Richard Horton, Editor of *The Lancet*, challenged the current performance indicators in an open letter to Ian Kennedy who chairs the Healthcare Commission – the body now responsible for the star-rating system and for whatever system will replace it.

The star ratings that you published and defended last week are having a damaging effect on the health service you and I care about. Worse still, they are likely to undermine public confidence in a health service that enjoys an unparalleled commitment from its doctors, nurses and allied health workers.

(Horton 2004: 401)

Horton went on to report on the demoralisation at one hospital that had lost a star, despite meeting seven of the nine key targets, including achieving shorter inpatient and outpatient waiting times, two-week maximum wait for all cancers, commitment to improving the working lives of staff and hospital cleanliness. The subsequent humiliation in the local press had served to further undermine staff morale and patient confidence. Questioning the validity and methodology of the star-rating system, Horton challenged Professor Kennedy to end the evaluations that he deemed as untrustworthy and unjust.

Changes to the evaluation system are being made and further changes are promised. It remains to be seen if they will serve as a more refined and fair tool. Meanwhile it is important for both staff and patients to be circumspect in how they interpret star ratings or any other performance data. They need to bear in mind that published figures and ratings only represent a snapshot in time, and may not be the most relevant criteria on which to judge the aspects of care that truly matter.

5 'Sorry' seems to be the hardest word

Revolving door

Susan glanced at her watch, and was surprised to discover that it had just gone four in the afternoon. Daniel was off sick from school, and she'd given him his lunch hours ago, but had not gotten around to having anything herself. She was in two minds as to whether to bother at this point, or to just have a cup of tea and a Mars bar and wait for supper. Despite the temptation, she smiled ruefully as she remembered the conversation she'd had the previous week with Dr Stebbing.

She'd been to see him because her blood pressure was running a bit high – a problem that had only come to light when she had finally had her routine smear, more than a year late. Dr Stebbing had made her promise to take better care of herself, to eat properly, lose weight and take some exercise. He'd listened sympathetically when she'd told him how difficult things were at the moment – what with Matthew being in and out of work and having to juggle her own job and look after the children. When she'd finished letting off steam he'd told her very firmly that if she let her own health slip off the bottom of the agenda, she wasn't going to be any use to any of them. She knew he was right, of course, and in her heart of hearts she also knew she was on a very short fuse – snapping at everyone unnecessarily and regretting it immediately afterwards.

She put her head round the door of Daniel's bedroom to see if he wanted a drink. He was absorbed in eliminating aliens from the screen of his PlayStation, and her enquiry was greeted with a dismissive grunt. Susan was often frustrated at the amount of time Daniel – now nine – could spend sitting in front of a PlayStation, when it took such an effort to keep him sitting in front his homework. However, on this occasion she took it as a sign that his temperature was probably down and was pleased that he wasn't as listless as he had been in the morning. She headed into the kitchen and set about assembling herself some quiche and salad.

In general, things had been going pretty well over the past few years. Daniel had needed relatively few admissions to hospital, and communication between the GP practice, the community team and St Michael's had been great. Susan had been able to give Daniel a bit more autonomy to manage his own treatment and had steeled herself not to be over-protective. A couple of months back, she had even felt confident enough to take Sara to Paris for three days for her birthday, leaving Matthew and his parents to hold the fort. They'd thought about going as a family, but Matthew didn't feel he could ask for the time off when he'd only been in his new job for a couple of months.

Susan worried about Sara – but then Matthew said she worried about everything. Sometimes she found it hard to know whether he was really immune to worry, or just didn't talk about it. Whatever he said, she knew that Sara was bright and that she shouldn't have done so badly in her A-levels, failing two and just scraping through the third. It was impossible not to wonder if she would have done better at school if it hadn't been for the time and emotion they expended on Daniel . . . and the tension that had put on their marriage.

The trip to Paris seemed like a distant dream now, because only a couple of weeks after they got back things had started to go badly downhill. Daniel had gone down with a chest infection, and when he was admitted to St Michael's they had found a bug called *Pseudomonas aeruginosa* in his lungs. Susan had been really frightened. She had read a lot about the kinds of bugs that infect children with cystic fibrosis, and she knew that almost all cystic fibrosis patients got *Pseudomonas* sooner or later. But she also knew that if Daniel got chronically infected with it, it would gradually damage his lungs. Dr Khan had been very reassuring and told her that they could get rid of it with a three-week course of two really strong antibiotics – one by nebuliser (a face mask that made the drug into a fine mist) and one by mouth. That had all gone very well, but Daniel had only been back at school for a couple of weeks when he had gone down with another infection. Susan didn't think he had been right since.

Right now, he had been off school for almost a week, having yet another course of intravenous antibiotics. Normally he would bounce back after a couple of days, but he seemed to be taking much longer this time, and his temperature was still swinging. Susan was grateful that she could look after him at home rather than having to have him into St Michael's every time. But the downside was that she had had so much time off work recently that she was sure she was going to lose her job soon.

Today she felt stretched to the limit. It seemed as if half the world had been in and out of the house. First Sian, the home tutor had dropped in to see if Daniel was up to doing any school work. She had quickly realised that he wasn't ready yet and had gone off with a promise to call in the following week. Then the community pharmacist had arrived with another batch of antibiotics. He hadn't even left when Jane, Daniel's physio had arrived, and Susan had spent a long time talking to her about how difficult Daniel was becoming about doing his physiotherapy. In fact, he was bad enough when he was well, but completely impossible when he was sick.

Her mother had appeared just as she was putting the washing in the machine and tidying the plates still left from breakfast. Susan's heart sank as she started to unload 'a few things to tempt Daniel to eat a bit' from her bag. She knew her mum meant well, but she didn't feel up to facing the hour-long argument that she knew would ensue. She wondered whether today's topic was going to be how Matthew was failing to provide adequately for his family, or why Susan wasn't pushing Sara to retake her A-levels.

When she was finally alone with Daniel again, she felt as though her front door had been replaced with a revolving door, like the one in the local department store. She put her belated lunch on a tray, sank gratefully into a chair in front on the television and allowed an afternoon quiz show to float in front of her eyes. She had taken three mouthfuls when the doorbell rang. This time it was Penny, the nurse from the children's home-care team. Susan greeted her with a brittle cheerfulness.

'Oh dear, bad timing?' Penny said, as she caught sight of Susan's half-eaten lunch.

'No, really, it's good to see you,' Susan replied, and went into the kitchen to make tea.

But Penny knew her too well and, as Susan was busying herself with the kettle and cups, Penny came up behind her, put her hand on her shoulder and asked how she was doing.

'Fine, absolutely fine,' she said and began to sob inconsolably.

On the edge

It was four days later, and Susan was putting some fresh clothes in Daniel's side locker at St Michael's. Things had moved fast after Penny arrived at the house. She had been up to have a look at Daniel, found that his portacath site was red and tender and concluded that he probably had an infection in or around his intravenous line. It had only taken a couple of calls to the GP surgery and St Michael's, and then he was on his way back in to hospital. Susan had felt a mixture of disappointment and overwhelming relief.

'You were talking about the big trip that you had planned to the

Caribbean, the last time we were in,' Susan said to Gita Joseph, the staff nurse, who had arrived to do Daniel's observations and give him his drugs. 'Did you have a good time?'

'Yes, it was great,' Gita said as she marked Daniel's temperature on his chart, noting with satisfaction that it had been down for over twenty-four hours now. 'I had two lovely weeks. Went with my parents to see dad's aunt. We just got back a couple of days ago, although it seems like a lifetime ago already.'

Gita only had half her attention on her conversation with Mrs Johnson. The ward was ridiculously busy, and they were two nurses down. She needed someone to go down to theatre with the child in the next room, and she wasn't sure who they could spare.

'That's nice. I might just go and give Sara a quick call . . . Unless . . .' Susan hesitated.

Gita said 'Oh do go off, why not have a cup of tea? Daniel will be fine with me.'

Susan hadn't spoken to Sara since the previous afternoon, and she wanted to know she was OK. She seemed to be out most nights with Greg, her new boyfriend, and she was sure that half the time that Sara was on the back of his bike he was over the limit.

Gita looked around for someone to check Daniel's antibiotics with her. There should always be two nurses checking a drug dose, but were no other qualified staff in sight, so she called one of the students over. She had a fleeting moment of doubt as she drew up the second syringe. It seemed like quite a large dose, but these children were often on whacking doses of amikacin when their lines were infected.

Daniel looked at the syringe too, and said 'It's a lot isn't it? More than I get at home . . .'

'Yes, I'm sure that's why we've managed to get your temperature down Daniel,' Gita said, as she dismissed her momentary concern and started the infusion.

Over the edge

The infusion had finished and Daniel was sitting up reading *Harry Potter* when Susan came back.

'You OK love?' she asked, walking across to the bed, ruffling the top of his head.

'Yep. Fine. You know what's funny though . . . I thought I was getting better, but I think they're giving me more of the antibiotic. It was a much bigger syringe than normal.'

'Oh, don't be silly, Daniel,' Susan said, picking up his drug chart. One thing about having nine years experience of parenting a child with cystic fibrosis – she knew her way around drug charts and doses. 'I'm sure it was just more diluted. They'd have told me this morning on the ward round if they were worried or were changing anything.' But as she opened his chart she saw immediately that he'd been given more than twice the previous day's dose.

David Storr, the Ward Registrar, confirmed that yes, there had been a mistake with the dose. But he said it 'wasn't much'.

Susan was furious. 'It was nearly two and a half times as much. You said so yourself. How can that be "not much"? The dose either matters or it doesn't matter. So what do you mean by "not much"?'

'Well, it's not a critical overdose or anything . . . but we will have to do some blood tests just to make sure it won't have any effect on his kidneys.'

'His kidneys?' Susan yelled at him. 'Christ, what's wrong with you people? You all tell me I need to get out more, to leave Daniel in your capable hands. Then when I leave him alone for a minute you pump him full of a drug that could damage his kidneys.'

'And as for her,' gesturing towards Gita, who had just come back into the room, 'she's not fit to be a children's nurse. Surely she should have known it was the wrong dose.'

Daniel started to cry. He was scared, because of having had too much medicine, because of the shouting. Because of what they said. No one noticed. He didn't want them to notice and quietly rubbed his nose on his sleeve.

'Mrs Johnson, please,' Dr Storr sounded calm but looked shaken. 'What I mean is that we'll need to monitor him, obviously, keep him in a few days for observation, but a mistake like this is really very unlikely to cause problems.'

Gita edged further into the room and gathered up the charts that Susan had thrown to the floor. 'Please Mrs Johnson . . . I understand how you must feel. How about if I get you a cup of tea, and maybe you'll feel a bit calmer?'

'A bit calmer?' Susan echoed, her voice rising again. 'A bit calmer?! I don't want to feel a bit calmer. I just want to know how the hell this happened.'

It wasn't my fault

David Storr felt a rising sense of panic and wondered if he should phone the Medical Defence Union. But that seemed a bit over the top for such a small error, and anyway he realised that the first person he should talk to was Dr Khan, his consultant. He was in clinic, but had been very reassuring over the phone. He had told him not to worry and that they'd talk about it properly when he got back to the ward. So, in the meantime, he decided to discuss it with Meena, one of the other registrars.

'Really, it wasn't my fault,' he said, trying to convince himself that this was true. 'I mean, I know I was the one who rewrote his drug chart this morning, but look . . . the bloody locum who wrote it up in the first place had such God-awful handwriting.' He thrust the previous drug chart under Meena's nose and said 'Wouldn't you have mistaken that 4 for a 9?'

Meena didn't say anything, because there wasn't any point. She knew this was a real classic: there was much more chance of making an error when doing something mindless like copying over information from a full drug chart to a fresh one than when writing up a drug from scratch. David went on, 'It was my first day back and that stupid locum had left me with a load of loose ends that he didn't sort out . . . unbooked tests, discharge summaries not written. I suppose I should have stopped to check Daniel's age, looked at his weight, maybe recalculated the dose . . . but who would do that when they were just reboarding a chart?'

There was a long silence while Meena tried to think what to say. David moved the mountain of unwritten discharge summaries to one side, sat heavily at the desk and said in a low undertone, 'I'm just so sorry I was in such a rush, so sorry that this has happened.'

'God, I'm so sorry that I didn't take more notice of Daniel,' Gita said to the ward sister, while she was filling out an incident form so that the events of the morning could be properly investigated. 'I should have realised immediately – that was a reasonable dose for a chunky twelve-year-old, not a scrawny nine-year-old. But it's not really my fault, surely – it was David who wrote up the wrong dose. And Daniel did have a severe line infection. The trouble is, they're such a difficult family to work with. They get aggressive at the drop of a hat, thinking they know best, helping themselves to stuff from the treatment room, reading the notes. It's almost like they expect us to screw up all the time, and now we have . . .'

Susan had been on the phone to Matthew for the past fifteen minutes. 'It would just help if one of them could say sorry, but they make it feel like I'm the one in the wrong. They're all giving me a wide berth, trying not to catch my eye when they come in and out of the room.

I don't know . . . maybe I shouldn't have picked that moment to leave him . . . and I'm sorry I yelled at them all. I know they're doing their best. That they're all really busy.

I just want him to be better, and I want not to be here, and I want to know that it's not our fault. My fault. I don't know how to do the right thing anymore . . .'

Daniel knew it was all his fault . . . but there was no one he could tell. He should have explained to Gita what he meant – that it was a bigger dose than yesterday and that he thought she had it wrong. Then maybe none of this would have happened.

But it wasn't just that. Really the whole thing was his fault. His fault for being ill, for having cystic fibrosis. If it wasn't for him, he was sure his Dad wouldn't keep losing his job, his Mum wouldn't be crying the whole time and Sara would have done better at school. Everyone seemed to be shouting at each other all the time . . . at home, in the hospital – and it was all because of him.

The door opened and someone new came in. She told him her name was Judy, and she was a play therapist. She looked over his shoulder at the picture he'd been drawing. It was a picture of a house and a garden, with lots of dead bodies on the front lawn and one small figure standing in the middle with a laser gun.

'Gosh, that's a pretty frightening picture,' Judy said, sitting on the edge of his bed. 'Want to tell me about it?'

Cut! Rewind

Daniel suffered a drug error – arguably a relatively trivial error – and he was very unlikely to come to harm as a result. So did it matter? Could it have been prevented? What should have been done to remedy the situation? Was someone to blame – and, if so, who?

As far as Susan was concerned, this should just never have happened. But as is often the case, the 'knock-on' effects from the error were probably far more damaging than the error itself. Daniel's misery, the blow to Susan's confidence in the team at St Michael's, and the impact on David Storr and Gita Joseph, who would both be left feeling wretched about their role in the affair.

At its simplest level, it would be easy to lay blame at the feet of David – who after all wrote the wrong dose on a drug chart – and on Gita, who might have been expected to spot that it was too large a dose for a child of Daniel's age and size. Surely the simplest course of action would be to reprimand or punish both of them, perhaps offer them some additional training to make sure they didn't make such an error again, and for all to move on? In fact, such a response would be of limited value in addressing this situation or in preventing a recurrence of the same problem.

As in previous chapters, situations are never as simple as they appear on the surface and, once again, analysis is at three levels. First, what was it about the immediate systems and processes that allowed such an error to occur? Second, how could the individuals involved have behaved differently – either in the run-up to the error or, just as importantly, in its aftermath? And, finally, what are the broader societal pressures and belief systems that determine how we respond to error and to those we perceive to be responsible?

THE HEALTH-CARE SYSTEM: UNDERSTANDING SYSTEM ERROR

By 2003, twenty-three patients worldwide had died or had been paralysed as a result of the cancer chemotherapy drug vincristine being accidentally injected into their spine rather than a vein (Donaldson 2002: 46). This is an example of how the same error can occur time and time again, although different staff and hospitals were involved on each occasion.

One of the most important reasons for trying to understand error causation is to prevent recurrences such as the vincristine example given above. James Reason, Emeritus Professor of Psychology in Manchester, has had a major role in developing understanding in the field and in moving thinking forward from a 'person approach' to a 'system approach' (Reason 2000: 768).

To err is human

> Fallibility is part of the human condition. We can't change the human condition, but we can change the conditions under which humans work.
>
> (Reason 2000: 768)

The person approach focuses on the actions of the people at the front line, with the aim of identifying countermeasures that can reduce human variability. Approaches ranging from punitive, such as disciplinary proceedings, and naming and shaming, to educational, such as improving information and retraining, are all designed to eliminate human error. None will ever succeed, because only a certain proportion of human error is amenable to such measures. Making mistakes is a part of the human condition and will never be completely eradicated.

Human error comes in a wide variety of shapes and forms, and the flow chart below demonstrates how different the causes can be:

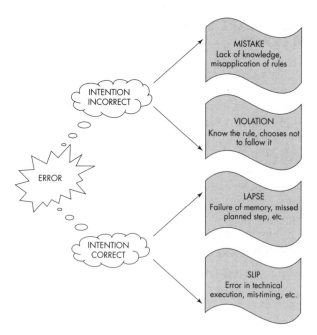

Figure 5.1 Classification of errors.

Intention incorrect

One major subgroup of errors occurs because the person sets out on
what transpires to be the wrong course of action (i.e., things went
according to plan, but the plan was wrong). These errors can either
be mistakes (through lack of knowledge about what to do, or through
misapplication of rules) or violations (the person knows the rule but
doesn't follow it). Sometimes there can be perfectly good reasons for
violating a rule, and this is why clinical guidelines are intended to be
just that: they should guide the clinician, but at some point an experienced judgement may need to be made in unusual circumstances.
And, sometimes, those judgements, made carefully and thoughtfully,
can be wrong. Equally, people sometimes know the rules but fail to
follow them because they're taking a short cut or are not motivated
to do things as they should.

Intention correct

The second subgroup occurs when the person sets off on a course of
action which, if they carried it though successfully, would culminate
in the right result, but something goes wrong in the process (i.e., good
plan, poor outcome). Where things go wrong in the execution, it is
called a 'slip'; where due to a failure of memory, a 'lapse'. 'Slips' and
'lapses' are more likely to occur through distraction, multitasking or
tiredness, and during routine or repetitive tasks.

As a general rule, junior doctors tend to make more errors of the
'intention incorrect' variety than senior doctors. They make these
'mistakes' through lack of experience, since they are less skilled at
interpreting and applying their knowledge and making the right plans.
For example, a very junior surgeon may make an error during an
operation because he is less knowledgeable about the right approach;
he makes a 'mistake' in how he tackles the task. By contrast, an experienced surgeon is unlikely to make such a 'mistake', but may cause a
similar error through a 'slip'. Of course, that is not to say that junior
doctors aren't also subject to 'slips' and 'lapses'.

What does all this mean in practice? In effect, it means that more
training, more supervision, more support and disciplinary procedures
can all help to eliminate mistakes that come about through inexperience, lack of knowledge, poor judgement or outright failure to follow
procedures. But errors due to 'slips' and 'lapses' will always occur –
and sometimes the best people make the worst errors.

So there has to be a safety net – a way to prevent these inevitable errors from turning into serious disasters for patients and families.

The Swiss cheese model

The 'system approach' is based on two fundamental premises. First, there is the self-evident reality that humans are fallible, as discussed above. Second, and more importantly from a prevention perspective, mishaps tend to fall into recurrent patterns. The same set of circumstances can result in the same errors, regardless of the people involved. The vincristine data referred to earlier is a classic example of this.

This predictability is heartening for those who seek to tackle the problem, because it means that by identifying error-prone situations, it is possible to take action to minimise risk. Examples of situations that are high risk are when people are tired, staffing is short and equipment is old or faulty. The first line of defence is therefore to try to plug these holes and rectify the weaknesses in the system – the so-called 'latent conditions'. Dr Storr wrote the wrong dose in the context of other problems or 'latent conditions': the poor handwriting of his locum colleague, a problem which will be largely solved when electronic prescribing is as widespread in hospital as in general practice; the very fact of having a locum covering in the first place, and the staff shortages that may have made this necessary (see Chapter 4); and the lack of continuity of care – neither David Storr nor Gita Joseph had been on duty the day before. In addition Daniel's large and disorganised set of notes – a common problem for long-term patients and another compelling driver for electronic patient records – would have made it harder for Dr Storr had he actually tried to check Daniel's antibiotic dose.

Apart from system changes that might have reduced the likelihood that Dr Storr would write up the wrong dose, other defensive layers could have been in place that might have 'captured' the error before it could result in harm. For example, the ward pharmacist might have spotted the error, so might Gita herself, or another nurse crosschecking the dose with Gita. And finally there was Daniel. Patients – even small ones – often know best.

The way in which defences, barriers and safeguards trap errors has been elegantly described in the Swiss cheese model of system accidents. In this model, the weaknesses in the system are conceptualised as the holes in each layer of cheese. Fortunately, individual holes do not normally matter because there are other layers in place. Problems

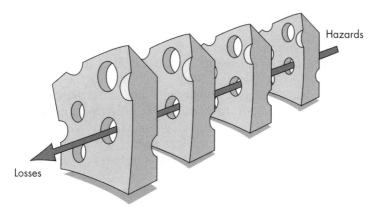

Figure 5.2 The Swiss-cheese model of error.

Source: Reason 2000. Reproduced with kind permission from BMJ Publishing Group.

only occur in the very unusual circumstance where all the holes line up (see Figure 5.2).

Even then, the vast majority of the errors that don't get 'trapped by the cheese', and that translate into a real event are relatively harmless. The wrong patient is given a paracetamol tablet, or someone has an extra blood test. But, once in a while, and once is always once too often – something very serious happens.

Box 5.1 Learning points for clinicians and patients: causes of errors

- As long as there are humans involved, there will always be errors. However, only a small minority of errors translate into an event that causes serious harm.
- Sometimes the best clinicians can make the worst mistakes.
- Mishaps are not random. They tend to occur in recurrent patterns.
- 'Latent conditions' – or weaknesses in the system – can often be identified and remedied before a serious adverse event occurs.
- Whether you are a clinician or a patient, you may be able to help prevent a future error by identifying and alerting someone to a weakness in the system.

An organisation with a memory

No hospital is immune to serious error and, sadly, in 1997 a child died at GOSH after vincristine was erroneously injected into his spine; he was one of the twenty-three cases cited in the above data. Following a detailed inquiry, 'latent conditions' and systemic problems were identified and addressed, and the inquiry report made thirty-two recommendations for change in pre-admission/communication, organisation of haematology/oncology theatre lists, hospital policies and prescribing, with special emphasis on cytotoxic drugs and staff training.

In cases such as these it is not enough for one institution to learn from a serious mistake. The learning needs to be shared across the NHS and more broadly. In the case of intrathecal[1] vincristine, a report produced in 2001 (Woods 2001) made recommendations about how to reduce intrathecal medication errors – by changing both systems and training. The recommendations included ensuring that intrathecal and intravenous cytotoxic drug treatments are given at different times, by different people and in different clinical locations – and by packaging vincristine in such a way that it can only be given through an intravenous line and cannot be injected into the spine.

This approach to learning from adverse events was launched in 2000 through a seminal report called *An Organisation with a Memory* (Department of Health 2000b). In his Foreword to the report, Alan Milburn said:

> Advances in knowledge and technology have [. . .] immeasurably increased the complexity of health care systems. Their unique combination of processes, technologies and human interactions means that modern health care systems are among the most complex in the world. With that complexity comes an inevitable risk that at times things will go wrong. And in health care when things go wrong the stakes are higher than in almost any other sphere of human activity.

The report highlights some thought-provoking statistics. For example, adverse events in which harm is caused to patients occur in 10 per cent of admissions to NHS hospitals. Although this statistic sounds alarming, it needs to be put in context. First, *serious* harm occurs in a

1 Into the spine

much smaller percentage of those cases. Second, hospital admissions are only the tip of the iceberg of NHS encounters (see Chapter 3), so do not represent the majority of clinical situations.

Nonetheless, high volumes inevitably mean more errors; for example, a 600-bed teaching hospital with 99.9 per cent error-free drug ordering, dispensing and administration will experience 4,000 drug errors a year. This means that mechanisms have to be in place to limit the adverse consequences of the errors that occur.

The conclusions of the report are outlined in the box below:

Box 5.2 Learning points for clinicians: conclusions of *An Organisation with a Memory*

- There must be unified mechanisms for reporting and analysis when things go wrong.
- There must be a more open culture, in which errors or service failures can be reported and discussed.
- There must be mechanisms for ensuring that, where lessons are identified, the necessary changes are put into practice.
- There must be a much wider appreciation of the value of the system approach in preventing, analysing and learning from errors.

So what has happened since this report – and has the number of errors reduced? The majority of clinicians would be confident in saying that there have been two closely related changes in culture and practice since the report: a reduced emphasis on individual blame and, following on from this, an increased emphasis on system improvement through enhanced reporting of critical incidents and near misses. These changes are not easy to develop and maintain and, despite good progress, there are still unresolved problems at all levels.

Eliminating blame culture

Research has shown that it is not just particular situations that are 'error prone'. Some institutions are more likely to generate errors, while others are 'high-reliability organisations'. High-reliability organisations operate on the expectation that errors will occur and that they need to train their staff to recognise and recover them. Conversely, institutions and systems with a poor track record have been shown to act as if errors are not to be expected and to blame individuals when they occur (Reason et al. 2001: ii21).

The 'retrospectoscope' – the lens through which we see the world with the power of hindsight – is a wonderful device that makes life a very black-and-white phenomenon. The paths and events that converged to precipitate a disaster can be seen with crystal clarity. With hindsight, there can be only one outcome – the one that happened – whilst for those who were involved there were multiple possible options and choices. Sidney Dekker (Dekker 2002) uses a tunnel analogy to describe how easy it is for those outside to see all the possible branch points, twists and exits, whilst those inside the tunnel are not afforded this oversight. Blame follows easily from this hindsight perspective.

Reducing the 'blame response' is fraught with difficulties. First, whatever the organisational response, there may well be censure and recrimination from a number of quarters: colleagues, seniors, patients and families and, most alarmingly, the media. Indeed, one of the ironies of *An Organisation with a Memory* (Department of Health 2000b) was that its launch was accompanied by headlines totally opposite in spirit from a central tenet of the report, blame reduction. Jane Smith, writing in the *BMJ* (Smith 2000: 1738), cited just some of these headlines: 'Warning System to Catch Shipmans and Ledwards set up by the NHS' (*Independent*); 'Early Warning System to Catch Bad Doctors' (*Guardian*); 'Warning System to Put the Spotlight on Killer Doctors' (*Express*). Since then, press reporting of medical errors has continued in much the same vein: 'She Was Killed by a Hospital' (*Evening Standard*, February 2001); 'Anger as Fatal Jab Doctor Freed' (*BBC News*, September 2003); 'Widow Awarded £800,000 for Doctor's Blunder' (*The Times*, July 2004). In almost all tragedy reporting by the press, whether in a medical setting or more broadly, there has to be a victim and a villain, and there is presently little sign of a more sophisticated media approach.

Secondly, and importantly in terms of both professional regulation and public confidence, 'no blame' cannot and should not mean that individuals can be absolved of appropriate professional responsibility (Walton 2004: 163). Thus a 'just' culture is perhaps a more appropriate aspiration than a 'no-blame' culture. Doctors, nurses and other clinical staff have an ethical, moral and professional obligation to be open and honest about errors. All clinicians ultimately have to be held to account for their actions.

Whilst difficult and traumatic, early disclosure has been shown to be less likely to result in litigation and press censure than delayed disclosure (Lamb 2004: 3), and it is the role of health-care organisations to support clinicians in taking this step. This requires staff to have a great deal of trust in their organisation. Firth-Cozens (2004: 56) has demonstrated how important organisational leadership is in developing this trust and how fragile a commodity it is.

Critical incident reporting; a miss is as good as a mile

The aim of reducing the blame culture is not just to encourage reporting of errors that result in serious harm. These are the tip of the iceberg, but equally important to system safety are the 'critical incidents', the less severe errors, the warning events and 'near misses'. Health care has not had to reinvent the wheel in developing systems for critical-incident reporting. There is a long tradition of this in the aviation industry, the military, the nuclear-power industry and many other commercial settings (Barach and Small 2000: 759). Reporting of minor incidents and near misses has the advantage that the stakes are lower and the numbers are greater, so it is easier to encourage active and safe engagement from clinicians.

Box 5.3 Learning points for clinicians: learning from errors

- All clinicians have a responsibility to report critical incidents and thus to contribute to organisational safety.
- If you are worried about reporting an error, particularly about issues of confidentiality, you can talk it through first with a colleague, a senior member of staff or a member of the Patient and Staff Safety team.
- Open discussion is important. As a senior member of staff, the ability to talk about your own previous errors with junior team members will provide them with a role model based on openness and honesty.
- Reflective learning is crucial. Keep a record in your portfolio of your learning from critical incidents and errors, whether your own or others.

Reporting of errors and critical incidents may help individual hospitals to identify local problems, but there also needs to be a way of collecting information nationally so that errors that occur in many different health-care settings can be tackled more effectively, as in the vincristine example described earlier. One important outcome of *An Organisation with a Memory* (Department of Health 2000b) was the formation of the National Patient Safety Agency (NPSA) in July 2001. The aim of the NPSA is to collate information about adverse incidents, to ensure that lessons are learnt from an analysis of these incidents and to develop solutions to systemic problems.

As to whether all these measures have reduced errors, it is very difficult to answer this question in an evidence-based manner. First, it is hard to collect representative and comprehensive data to compare two points in time and, second, technology moves on, so that the complexities referred to by Alan Milburn intensify. At the same time, service-delivery models evolve and change. But, perhaps most importantly, once our culture makes error-reporting possible, the immediate effect is an apparent rise in errors, not because more are occurring, but because of greater openness. Fortunately, national systems for recording and monitoring errors and near misses are becoming more sophisticated, and the NPSA has now set up a National Reporting and Learning System (NRLS) which is the first of its kind in the world. The NRLS will enable health-service organisations to electronically collate information in a standard format so that in time it will be possible to analyse trends and patterns much more effectively and to answer some of these complex questions.

THE SOCIETAL CONTEXT: NO FAULT COMPENSATION?

In a system that can never be error free, it is inevitable that some patients will suffer substantial harm as a result of the health care they receive. From a societal perspective it is just that they should be compensated. But who should compensate them? The doctor? The hospital? The Government? And how should the compensation be managed? Should patients who have suffered a misfortune through no fault of their own be expected to fight for fair recompense? Or should all patient claims be assumed to be justified? And, if so, what about the potential for abuse and the cost to the NHS?

A number of countries (Denmark, Finland, Sweden and New Zealand) have opted for such a 'no-fault' compensation scheme, either for all forms of injury howsoever caused (New Zealand) or confined to the medical sphere (Sweden). New Zealand's Accident Compensation Corporation <http://www.acc.co.nz> came into being in 1974 and now provides for and manages compensation for any accident. It is also closely involved in work on accident prevention. Much discussion has centred on the feasibility of such a scheme here, and it has many advocates who believe that it could be successful.

Clinical negligence

Clinical negligence claims operate under an area of civil law called 'tort' law. A tort is an act or omission that causes harm – in this context, to an individual. In order to be able to win a case of negligence a person must be able to prove three things: first, that he or she was owed a duty of care; second, that the duty was breached; and finally that he or she suffered injury or harm that was caused by the breach in duty. In a hospital, a doctor owes such a duty if he or she has undertaken responsibility for the care of a patient.

The standard of care: the Bolam test

'The Bolam case' (*Bolam v. Friern Barnet Hospital Management Committee*, 1957) was a landmark case in setting legal precedent in relation to medical negligence for the next forty years. In 1954, John Bolam had electro-convulsive therapy for depression, during which he was not given any form of relaxant or manual restraint, nor was he given any warning about the risks of the treatment. He sustained dislocated hips and a fractured pelvis. When the case came to court in 1957, it went against the plaintiff on the basis of Justice McNair's direction to the jury:

> A doctor is not guilty of negligence if he has acted in accordance with practice accepted as proper by a responsible body of medical men skilled in that particular art. Put another way, a man is not negligent if he is acting in accordance with such a practice just because there is a body of opinion that would take a contrary view.
> (Lord Justice McNair in *Bolam v. Friern Hospital Management Committee*, 1957)

The judgment was notable because it meant that the medical profession could, in effect, set the standards. Those standards, by definition, were not based on evidence-based best practice ('a man need not possess the highest expert skill'), making it possible to legitimise quite marginal practices. For example, in *Maynard v. West Midlands Health Authority*, 1985, the Bolam principle was upheld even though medical opinion was divided. The fact that there was a body of opinion that supported the defendant's actions was enough to overturn the negligence claim, even though other responsible clinicians gave a different view.

The principle was applied not only to diagnosis (*Maynard v. West Midlands Health Authority*) and treatment (*Whitehouse v. Jordan*, 1981), but also to the level of information that was disclosed to a patient (*Sidaway v. Board of Governors of the Bethlem Royal Hospital and the Maudsley Hospital*, 1985). In this latter case, a patient underwent an operation that carried a very slight risk of spinal injury. Although the operation was properly performed, her spine was injured and she was badly disabled. By today's standards, it was clear that consent was not properly informed but, on the Bolam test, the practice met standards of the time. A further case (*Wilsher v. Essex Area Health Authority*, 1988) established that the same standards were expected, regardless of the seniority or experience of the doctor.

A final important distinction is that the Bolam test is based on what was actually done. In negligence cases generally, the test is a normative test based on what should have been done, and judgment is set against that benchmark. This has made it more difficult for plaintiffs to succeed in medical negligence cases and was commented on by the Pearson Commission, who noted the difference between the success of negligence claims generally (60–80 per cent) as opposed to medical negligence claims (30–40 per cent) (Jones 2000: 237).

Harm and causation: advent of Bolitho

A move from Bolam was finally effected through *Bolitho v. City and Hackney Health Authority* (1997) (Samanta and Samanta 2003: 443). Patrick Bolitho was a two-year-old boy with croup who eventually died having suffered severe brain damage as a result of a cardiac arrest. The case revolved around the question of whether the outcome was due to a lack of intervention by the paediatrician, who failed to attend him and put a tube into his airway to help him breathe. Although the doctor had conceded that it had been negligent not to attend the child when called, she argued that even if she had gone she would not have intubated him. She had expert witnesses who supported her claim that non-intubation was a clinically justifiable response. The plaintiff had differing expert evidence – that a reasonably competent doctor would have intubated in those circumstances and that therefore the doctor ought to have done so.

Patrick Bolitho's mother lost the case in the High Court and in the Court of Appeal. In the House of Lords (the highest court in England and Wales, where five Law Lords give judgement), the judges finally reinterpreted the Bolam test. They ruled that it was not sufficient that a body of opinion supported the doctor's actions – the court had to be satisfied that that body of opinion was logical. Despite this, the case for the plaintiff still failed on grounds of causation, because the court accepted the view that it was logical not to intubate. Nonetheless, the case was a landmark, since for the first time it was deemed a matter for the court, and not medical opinion, to decide the standard of professional care.

> The court has to be satisfied that the exponents of the body of opinion relied upon can demonstrate that such opinion has a logical basis. In particular, in cases involving, as they so often do, the weighing of risks against benefits, the judge before accepting a body of opinion as being responsible, reasonable or respectable, will need to be satisfied that, in forming their views, the experts have directed their minds to the question of comparative risks and benefits and have reached a defensible conclusion on the matter.
>
> (Lord Browne-Wilkinson in *Bolitho* v. *City and Hackney Health Authority*, 1997)

Responsibility of the hospital

The provisions that apply in proving negligence by individual doctors are true for the hospital itself, which is vicariously liable for the acts of its staff. Furthermore, the hospital also has a responsibility to ensure that there are appropriate systems in place for its staff to follow. This was demonstrated in the case of *Robertson* v. *Nottingham Health Authority* (1997). The plaintiff was a child with severe cerebral palsy, and her case was that her disability was caused as a result of asphyxia (oxygen starvation) during labour. It was demonstrated that during the labour there had been a breakdown in communication between the doctor and the nursing staff and that, as a result, medical instructions had not been carried out. The hospital was found to be at fault because there was no evidence before the court as to the systems in place for ensuring avoidable breakdown of communication. However, as with *Bolitho*, the plaintiff's case failed on the issue of causation. Nonetheless, had causation been proven, the hospital would have been liable on the basis of system failure, even though none of its staff were considered to have acted negligently.

Negligence claims are costly to the NHS, and in 1995 the NHS Litigation Authority was established to handle such claims against NHS bodies in England. In 2003–4, 422.5 million pounds was paid out in connection with clinical negligence claims. This figure includes both damages paid to patients and legal costs. NHS trusts fund these claims by paying into the Clinical Negligence Scheme for Trusts (CNST) which, like any other insurance scheme, provides a lower premium to lower risk organisations. CNST sets rigorous safety standards which trusts have to meet in order to qualify for the lower premiums, so this is a powerful incentive to improve local systems and processes and, hence, to reduce error. Encouragingly, the number of clinical negligence claims dropped by 20 per cent between 2002–3 and 2003–4.

Making amends

Despite some of the case-law changes described above, medical-negligence claims remain protracted, acrimonious and traumatic for all concerned. Lord Woolf, in his report in 1996, found that 78 per cent of medical-negligence cases were settled after the majority of the expense had been incurred (Otton 2001: 72). In 2003, the Chief Medical Office launched a consultation document on an alternative system for compensating patients (Donaldson 2003). The option of a full no-fault scheme was rejected on the basis of cost and its potential for abuse. However, a fast-track system for small claims (up to 30,000 pounds) is proposed, alongside delivery of a package of care providing remedial treatment. Specific provisions for children who suffer neurological damage as a result of birth injury are also proposed.

At time of writing, there has not yet been a conclusion to the consultation, although the proposed scheme has come in for criticism from those who think it will increase the number of claims, put an additional burden on clinicians and managers, and still not reduce protracted claims culminating in excess legal costs (Capstick 2004: 457).

Part of the problem lies in the issue of who is deserving of compensation and why. The consultation document gives a cogent account of why, under the current system, both patients and clinicians suffer as a result of the stress and trauma engendered by litigation. The proposed NHS Redress Scheme is therefore aimed at compensating those who have been harmed as a result of seriously substandard NHS hospital care. Patients would be eligible for payment for serious shortcomings in NHS care if the harm could have been avoided and if the adverse outcome was not the result of the natural progression of the illness. This is not a 'no-fault' compensation scheme, but one in which the nature of the fault is changed and is more broadly attributable. In identifying 'substandard' practice, there is also an implication of the option to benchmark standards against best practice, which is a very significant step forward from *Bolam* and *Bolitho*.

However, the proposals raise a whole new set of moral questions. In 1980, in relation to *Whitehouse* v. *Jordan* (1981), Lord Denning expressed the view that an error of judgement in a professional context did not amount to negligence. To test this, he said, 'One might ask the average competent and careful practitioner: "Is this the sort of mistake that you yourself might have made?" If he says: "Yes, even doing the best I could, it might have happened to me", then it is not negligent.' Although Lord Denning's view did not become law, Jon Holbrook (2003a) argues that if an error of judgement does not equate to negligence, then there is no moral culpability or stigma. If this is the case, then what is the justification for compensating someone whose child was damaged as a result of an error of judgement that any competent doctor could have made, and not compensating someone with an equally disabled child whose condition was genetically or congenitally determined? For that matter, why is it justified to compensate someone whose child was damaged as a result of irrefutable negligence, whilst not compensating someone with a similarly disabled child arising from a genetic condition or a blameless household accident? In practice, it could become very difficult to define an ethically defensible boundary to these proposals.

AT THE FRONT LINE: DEALING CONSTRUCTIVELY WITH COMPLAINTS

No matter how sophisticated our understanding of medical error and its precipitants, this is of limited value to the patient who suffers pain or discomfort as a result, or to the bereaved family in the tragic event that an error proves fatal. Families may be able to forgive, but it is harder to excuse and impossible to forget.

Whatever the explanation of the drug error in this scenario, one of the major failings was in the subsequent interaction with Susan and Daniel. In the aftermath of the error, everyone was sorry – both for the error itself and for the part they had played in it. They all managed to say so, but not to each other!

'Sorry' seems to be the hardest word

Being open about a mistake and saying 'sorry' at the earliest opportunity is one of the most important responses to error. Frequently, an acknowledgement that an error has occurred and an apology is what the patient most needs to hear, closely followed by an explanation of how the error occurred. These things do not undo what has happened, but they can go some way towards restoring trust or at least avoiding the development of greater mistrust.

Bea Teuten, PALS Advocate at GOSH, describes how patients are often treated in the aftermath of an error. Phrases such as 'We were treated like lepers', 'Everyone tried to avoid eye contact with us', 'No one spoke to us', 'It was as though it was all our fault', 'Everyone suddenly became falsely cheerful', all sum up the understandable but dysfunctional staff responses that can result from embarrassment and guilt.

In this scenario, Gita Joseph and David Storr needed to sit down with Susan and, after apologising, they needed to explain what steps would be taken to look after Daniel and to deal with any impact on him. They also needed to explain the steps that would be taken to investigate how the situation had occurred. In the immediate aftermath of an error the reasons for the problem are often unclear, and a fuller investigation of events is generally necessary. Patients are able to understand and accept this, provided they are told how this is going to be managed, who will feed back to them and when. Allocating a member of the team, preferably someone senior, to maintain proactive communication with the family is of the utmost importance. In this scenario, Dr Khan would probably be the best person to follow things up with the family. Given how distressed Susan was, it would probably have been better to talk to her separately from Daniel in the first instance, but there was a self-evident need to then go and talk things through with Daniel and to reassure him.

Balancing the need to give an apology against fear of litigation is a difficult dilemma for clinicians. However, an apology is not an admission of liability, and, paradoxically, clinicians may increase the likelihood of litigation by failing to apologise at an early stage. For example, in 1995 (Lamb 2004), a patient in New Zealand had a late diagnosis of cervical cancer because of problems in the cervical-screening process and reporting of results. Ultimately this went to court, and the legal battle continued until 2003 when a settlement with the retired pathologist and the Crown was reached. The problems that were uncovered led to improvements in the national cervical-screening programme. Shortly before the settlement, the patient said that her response would have been entirely different if she had received an early apology and an assurance that there would be some planned remedial action to prevent a recurrence of this problem for other women. This case highlights two points: first, that after an apology and an explanation, patients often want to know that there will be some change to the system so that at least some good comes out of their misfortune and that other patients are spared similar suffering; and second, that a single individual can make a difference and can have an impact on systems and processes.

Conflict resolution the proactive way

One of the most important aspects of dealing with conflict is to be as proactive as possible in trying to resolve the issues before they escalate into a complaint or litigation. Unless patients have suffered serious harm, possibly associated with significant financial consequences, they are unlikely to want to engage in acrimonious complaints and litigation. Understandably, what they do want is a just resolution to their problem and some assurance that systems will be improved in future. Some examples of proactive conflict management, adapted from real cases at GOSH, are given below:

Taking patient concerns seriously

The problem

A child came back from surgery after a procedure that had brought to light complications from a previous operation. The parents felt that they should have been warned of these complications, while the ward found the parents extremely angry and thought them dishonest, refusing to believe their view that they had not been alerted to the possible complications. The parents felt their only option was litigation.

Resolution

An impartial member of the hospital staff took on a very proactive role in looking into the family's issues and listening to their version of events. This involved daily phone calls at a time convenient for the family and a visit to their home (since they had other young children) at their convenience. She discovered that the family were in fact correct in stating that they had never been warned of the complications (none had been identified on the consent form). A meeting was held with the consultant to discuss a set of questions drawn up by the family and shown to the consultant before the meeting. At the meeting the family had a chance to explain how traumatised they had felt, when 'everything had gone wrong', and how abandoned by the ward staff who had not spent time with them discussing the consequences. A number of system errors were identified (for example, an incorrect consent form) and agreement was reached as to what the hospital needed to do to address this. Minutes of the meeting detailed a timetable of agreed actions for the hospital and an update was sent to the family six months after the event so that they could be assured that the hospital had delivered on its promises.

Agreeing a joint action plan with the help of a third party

The problem

A family who had been regular patients at the hospital felt that they were being let down every time they came in to the ward. They felt that junior doctors did not appreciate the wealth of knowledge they had gained over the many years of managing their child's condition and that they were treated as though they had nothing constructive to say at consultations. The staff, on the other hand, saw the parents as demanding, rude and aggressive and felt that they treated the ward as a second home, inciting other parents to complain and never giving the staff a chance to get it right. Events escalated on one admission to the point that the junior doctor threw a cup at the father whilst the mother threatened to take the child away despite his need for surgery.

Resolution

The presence of an experienced and impartial member of staff enabled each party to discuss their issues separately. An agreed plan of action for future admissions was then put in place setting out the responsibilities for both staff and family alike. If ever serious issues arose again, the parties went back to discuss the issues and to revisit the care plan. This was a win–win situation for all: a long and acrimonious complaint was avoided and a positive way forward was found by all. The parents wanted the best for the child, as did the staff.

Some of the key principles of active conflict management are outlined below but, in addition, training courses can be very helpful and are widely available:

Box 5.4 Learning points for staff: proactive conflict resolution

- When a family or a child is unhappy about an aspect of care, concerns must be met constructively and respectfully. They may feel that the only way forward is an official complaint, but alternative approaches may be more beneficial for all. Hospitals and trusts have support systems for advising family and staff on these.
- If you need to meet parents or children to discuss problems, make sure they can attend easily – for example, do not arrange meetings at school pick-up time or at short notice.
- Despite your best intentions, you are at risk of entering discussions with a preconception that your systems and processes are right and that the family is wrong. An impartial third party can be very helpful in giving an objective view.

---

continued

- Where appropriate, offer the family the support of the PALS team. Consider whether you need a member of PALS or Patient and Staff Safety teams present at meetings with the family.

- Do not meet anger with anger. A parent's or patient's anger at a specific time may be justified. Put yourself in their shoes. The event that sparked the anger may have been the last straw. You need to defuse the situation with calm.

- Ensure that you have listened to and understood the family's concerns. Accept strong feelings and do not downplay them. Try to understand why the patient or parent feels as they do and show empathy, reflecting back that you have understood.

- If you made a mistake, apologise. And don't forget to apologise to the child if they are old enough to understand the situation. Saying 'sorry' is not an admission of liability, but recognises a problem. You are not saying 'I'm sorry, it's my fault' but 'I'm sorry this happened'.

- Where possible, give a full, frank explanation of what went wrong and, if appropriate, discuss steps that have been put in place to prevent it from happening again.

- Make a note of what is said, and what action patients or parents want you to take. Agree on this and provide contact details of who the family should get in touch with if they need further information. Copy to all who were present.

- If possible, do what the family asks of you. If not, explain clearly why not, discuss alternatives, agree the next best thing, and act on this.

- Make sure you do what you said you would do when you said you would do it. If you can't, contact the patient or family to explain what is going on and that you haven't forgotten about them.

- All too often, once the immediate fear of litigation or a more formal complaint fades, staff no longer see the necessity to follow through on these issues. Remember that for a family that has been badly let down and whose trust has been broken, a further lack of commitment to tackle the problems will almost inevitably rekindle the family's anger and lead to more formal litigation.

- Families often want to know what has happened to the specific staff member involved (for example, have they been disciplined, suspended, and so on). Although this is under-standable, staff have rights of confidentiality that should not be breached. Take further advice from your director of human resources if this causes difficulties.

- Consider whether it is possible to involve the family in service improvement. Actively seeking input from recipients demonstrates that their voices will be heard and this can help build their confidence in services that they receive.

Expert patients and parents

A further factor in Susan's situation was that she had become an 'expert parent' – skilled in the management of her child's condition and sometimes knowing more about the medical aspects than the professionals involved in his care. The same issue was a cause of tension in the second real-life scenario, outlined above.

Management of long-term illness is an increasingly important component of health care. As a result, much has been written about expert patients and their role in managing their own chronic illnesses. The Government is now launching a formal Expert Patient Programme to make best use of patients' expertise, both in self-management and in supporting others. Considerably less has been written about expert parents, although this is obviously equally important in paediatric conditions. Sometimes conflict arises when staff do not recognise or acknowledge the expertise of patients and families, as in the scenario illustrated above. As a result, they can feel threatened by expert patients or parents, especially if they are inexperienced or more junior (Kirk and Glendinning 2004: 209). Sometimes it is easier for a more secure, senior member of staff to admit that they don't know something than for a more junior member of staff to do so. They fear losing credibility but, in fact, admitting to limitations is more likely to engender trust and a good working relationship.

Formal complaints

Sometimes informal resolution fails, and it is important to be aware of the formal mechanisms for dealing with complaints:

Box 5.5 Learning points for clinicians and patients: stages in complaint resolution

- New legislation on management of NHS complaints came into force on 30 July 2004. Details of the complaints procedure can be found through the Department of Health web site <http://www.dh.gov.uk> or the NHS web site <http://www.nhs.uk>.
- Local resolution is always the primary goal.
- Should local resolution fail, the Healthcare Commission is now the responsible body for conducting an independent review.
- Finally, it is possible to appeal to the Health Service Ombudsman, who is independent of the NHS and the Government.

Box 5.6 Learning points for patients: making a formal complaint

- Make sure you have full details of the events you are complaining about: dates, times and, if appropriate, individuals. All this will save time and will ensure you have the facts to hand.
- Put your letter into headings; all too often the main issue of the complaint is eclipsed by a very long list of small things that have gone wrong.
- Always address your letter to the Chief Executive. You can always call the hospital switchboard to get the details.
- Place your, or your child's, hospital number as a main heading. If you don't know it, put the name and date of birth.
- Make clear what kind of redress you are seeking. Do you want a formal apology? Do you want to see what steps have been taken to ensure the event cannot happen again? Do you want to have a meeting? Do you want to be involved in developing the service for future users?
- Make a note in your diary of the day you sent the letter and keep a copy. You should receive a formal acknowledgement

within two working days and the formal written response within twenty.

- Don't forget that complaints need to be made within six months of the event.
- You can get free help in writing a complaint or with English from ICAS (Independent Complaints Advocacy Service) at <http://www.adviceguide.org.uk> or from the hospital's PALS.
- Filing a written complaint does not prevent you from bringing legal action. In some cases the hospital's detailed investigation will form the basis of an assessment of whether you will be eligible for legal aid.

Box 5.7 Learning points for patients: access to medical records

If you need to access your records in the aftermath of an error or because you have concerns about your treatment, the following guidance may be helpful:

- Patients can apply to see their full notes, and Department of Health policy is that this should be allowed subject to certain exemptions or compelling reasons to the contrary.
- Patients should apply in writing or electronically to the relevant 'data controller': their GP or the records manager at a hospital. Some health-care providers have standard request forms for this purpose.
- Patients don't need to say why they want access to their notes and should be helped to understand technical terms if necessary.
- Up to 10 pounds can be charged for access to computer records, and 50 pounds for copies of manual records, but patients can reduce costs by specifying which parts of notes they want to see.
- An explanation should be given if notes cannot be provided to a patient within forty days of their request.
- Access to information can be denied or limited if full access

continued

would cause physical or mental harm to the patient, to someone else, or would reveal information about a third party who has not given consent.
- If some information is withheld, patients do not have to be told, or told why.
- Those with parental responsibility can apply to see children's notes. Such access may be denied if health professionals do not think it would be in the child's best interests, or if the child is old enough to be asked consent and does not give it.

Aggressive or 'unlikeable' patients

> I've only been hit once in the line of duty. I didn't see it coming and it landed plum on the middle of my chin. The aggressor was seventy-five and female, and didn't quite pack enough power to floor me. She was the wife of a diabetic man who'd fallen over after an early morning hypo.[1] I cut his evening insulin and his sugar went the other way, causing him to fall over again. All my fault, of course.
>
> (Dr Phil Hammond, GP and broadcaster, 2003)

Given the events of the preceding weeks, Susan had clearly been about to snap, and the drug error was the final straw – precipitating a reaction that may have appeared unduly aggressive and volatile to the staff, but was entirely understandable given her situation. When confronted with an angry patient or parent, it is important that staff do not respond in similar vein.

It is equally important to acknowledge that whilst a large number of complaints are valid, are justified and are important drivers for system improvement, complainants can also be verbally or physically aggressive to staff. The Department of Health and the National Audit Office have reported year-on-year increases in attacks on NHS staff, despite the fact that many incidents are not reported. A majority of

---

1 Episode of low blood sugar, which can cause problems for diabetic patients.

these attacks are against front-line staff, for example in A&E departments, and are not necessarily in the context of a complaint about management or treatment. However, when aggressive behaviour is manifest in the context of a complaint, it is important to maintain a balance between protecting staff and continuing to address what might be a valid underlying grievance.

If a complainant is abusive or threatening, it is reasonable to require him or her to communicate only in a particular way – say, in writing and not by telephone – or solely with one or more designated members of staff, but it is not reasonable to refuse to accept or respond to communications about a complaint, until it is clear that all practical possibilities of resolution have been exhausted.

In response to the problem of escalating violence against NHS staff and a few very tragic fatalities, the NHS has adopted a zero-tolerance policy to aggressive or violent behaviour, making explicit that such behaviour will not be accepted. Individual trusts should have clear policies in place for managing this and should offer targeted training to staff in high-risk situations.

At the end of the day

'So what do you think then?' Ashok said again, an edge of irritation creeping into his voice.

'Sorry? Think about what?' Meena replied, dropping the paper she was reading onto the coffee table and trying to refocus her attention.

'About asking Jim and Katy over next weekend. Meena, what's the matter with you? You haven't heard a word I've said all evening.'

'Hmm, yes, sorry, I've been a bit distracted.'

'So I noticed. Are you going to tell me what's bugging you? Because if not, I'm going to bed.'

Meena spent some time looking into the dregs in her coffee mug, knowing that Ashok would patiently wait her out. 'Well actually, I'm feeling a bit guilty,' she said eventually. 'You remember that guy David Storr? The very jumped-up Mr Know-It-All who's just rotated into St Mike's from one of the London teaching hospitals?'

Ashok acknowledged that yes, he did remember her mentioning David.

'Yes, well, today he messed up rewriting a prescription chart for one of the chronic kids on the ward, and the kid got an overdose. His mum went ballistic.'

'Was the kid alright?'

'Yes, fine. It wasn't very serious. But it was the first time I've seen David phased about anything, and he came into the office to cry on my shoulder.'

Ashok still couldn't see where this was leading. 'Yes, so?'

'Well, to tell you the truth, I just felt rather pleased that it had happened to him. I was pretty unsympathetic. I can't stand the guy, and I couldn't think of anything to say that wouldn't let him know I was thinking "serves you right." Then I thought "What a bitch. There but for the grace of God go I".'

'So that's it? The reason for an evening of silence?'

'Well, no, not entirely. You see I was reading a paper the other day which says that some personality types are fundamentally more risky than others. Some of the information comes from other groups – aviation and the like – but it probably also translates to medicine. It was fairly predictable stuff – things like being a sensation-seeking, Type A personality, with high self-esteem, very little risk awareness and unwarranted confidence in your own abilities.[1]

'Well, it sounds as if you should do some kind of personality assessment when you select people for medical school and get rid of these characters at the outset. Then you could make health care a much safer business.'

'No, I think that'd be completely the wrong thing to do. The article talks about that as a possibility . . . but just think about it. On that basis you've probably just rejected the next generation of Christiaan Barnards and Robert Winstons.'

Ashok wondered fleetingly if that would be any bad thing, since he found Robert Winston profoundly irritating whenever he popped up on the television. He tried another tack. 'OK, I take that point. But from what you say, the article sums up your friend David Storr pretty well. Sounds as if he was an accident waiting to happen. It'll probably do him good to discover he's not God after all. In fact, he's bloody lucky it wasn't a serious mistake.'

'Ash, that's not actually the point. The thing is, although it was David today, it could be me tomorrow. In fact it was me yesterday. Well, not literally, but I mean I've made a few errors in my time. Written up a wrong drug which got picked up by the ward pharmacist . . . mislabelled a blood sample so that the wrong patient got treated for a low blood count. I mean, none of them were serious . . . but they could have been. I've just been lucky.'

---

1 The paper Meena was reading was Firth-Cozens et al. 2003: i16.

Ashok realised too late that he'd walked straight into this one. He should have realised earlier that this whole thing was obviously not about David Storr's error. It was about Meena's. He decided that he might as well work on the premise that nothing he said this evening was going to be right.

'Yes, well, you've always known that if you make a mistake at work, it's a much higher-stake business than mine. People are harder to replace than computer components. So why has this suddenly got to you now? You hardly fit the risky-doctor profile you've just told me about, so on statistical grounds, you'll probably be all right.'

'Well, that's easy for you to say, but it doesn't work like that. More and more doctors are being referred to the GMC, even though the majority end up being exonerated eventually. But think of the stress of that in the meantime. And did you know that seventeen doctors were charged with manslaughter in the 1990s? D'you think they deserved to go to prison for making a mistake at work? To lose their jobs and their livelihoods?'

'I don't know Meena. I guess it rather depends on what they'd done.'

'OK, I'll give you an example. A junior surgeon is doing a routine operation that should be well within his capabilities. Suddenly, there's an unexpected complication. He's never dealt with something like this, but he decides to wing it, to try and cope with it himself, rather than calling the consultant. The patient dies. Is he responsible?'

'Yes, of course. He should have called for help.'

'OK, agreed on that one. Now, what about this. He tries to get hold of his boss, but she's tied up doing another op. So he soldiers on, same result.'

'Well, that's different. Same result for the patient, but very different circumstances for him. I'd say that's not his fault.'

'Fine. So now, he thinks he can manage the emergency OK, because he's done a couple before under supervision, but not alone. He's obviously not as experienced as his consultant, but he knows she's been up operating all night, and decides to press on and not call her. Same result.'

'God Meena, I don't know. Should he have been more aware of his limitations? That's a difficult one. We're back to your risky-doctor profile. But in the real situation wouldn't there always be other people around he could talk to who might help him decide?'

'Well, I suppose that's true. Most of the time there are other people you can ask.'

'But, Meena, you haven't answered my question. Why are you so uptight about this all of a sudden? This isn't about David Storr, is it?' And suddenly he realised that he'd still missed the point. 'This isn't even about the trivial errors that you've made in the past, is it? Meena, what's wrong?'

Meena's face fell. 'It's Dad. He's been referred to the GMC because of a complaint against him. It was to do with a child-protection case he was involved in. I promised him I wouldn't tell you, but I couldn't help it. I just don't know what to do. He's so depressed about it, and Mum says he's talking about taking early retirement. But he's such a good doctor, and his work is his life now we've all left home.'

Ashok crossed the room and gave her a hug because it was hard to know what else to do. Her father, a paediatrician in Hartlepool, had been a role model for Meena all her life. Regardless of the rights and wrongs of the situation – of which he obviously knew nothing – it was going to be a stormy road ahead for all of them, watching this proud man go through the mill with the GMC and then dealing with the fall-out – whatever that might be.

UNRESOLVED QUESTIONS: LIABILITY FOR MANSLAUGHTER

In 2000, Ferner published a paper on the number of doctors charged with manslaughter as a result of fatal medical errors (Ferner 2000: 1212). This rose from only seven between 1867 and 1989 to seventeen between 1990 and 2000. The theme was picked up by Jon Holbrook, in an editorial in the *BMJ* in 2003 (Holbrook 2003b: 1118), in which he cited the circumstances culminating in a custodial sentence for Feda Mulhem, the registrar who instructed his junior to inject vincristine into the spine of Wayne Jowett. Internationally this was the twenty-third such error of its kind culminating in the paralysis or death of a patient.

> I know it's a lame excuse, but I am a human being.
> (Feda Mulhem 2003)

Holbrook compared the previous century's concept of gross negligence in a medical setting, 'if there was only the kind of forgetfulness which is common to everybody . . . it would be wrong to proceed against a man criminally in respect of such injury', with the more explicit criminalisation of fatal medical errors over the past decade. Societal attitudes have changed and, despite the rationale described earlier in this chapter for reducing blame culture, there is nonetheless a strong demand for culpability to be established, whether in relation to train crashes or medical errors.

Holbrook's questioning of the use of the criminal-justice system to punish Dr Mulhem, who, as he pointed out, was not seeking to harm Wayne Jowett but rather to further his recovery, produced a welter of responses from readers. Those supporting the action of the courts argued that killing someone on the road through a split second error of judgement would be just as likely to result in a criminal conviction of the motorist, despite a similar lack of intent to harm. Why, therefore, should the same standards not be applied to doctors? Lutchman (2003) reinforced this line of argument, making the point that the lack of intention to harm is not, in fact, mitigating, since it is the key defining feature of involuntary manslaughter (of which 'manslaughter by gross negligence' is one kind). Thus Mulhem's 'crime' was not his intent, but his mistake. He then went on to describe as 'misguided' the view that doing one's best is all that matters or is required or that inexperience, tiredness and overwork are adequate excuses.

Within the many responses supporting Holbrook's view, there was an important question raised as to how a culture that supports openness, honesty and the reporting of critical incidents can be developed in a climate in which those reporting the incidents are increasingly fearful of litigation. A heartfelt reply to Lutchman (2003), from a junior doctor, asked 'If "doing my best" isn't acceptable to society, then what is? If the law expects more then the law is wrong' (Psirides 2003).

Perhaps in considering the punishment meted out to Mulhem, it is apposite to consider what purpose a custodial sentence is intended to serve. First, it is supposed to deter offenders from repeating their crime – hardly applicable in this case since there was not an intent to criminal action in the first instance. Second, it is supposed to protect the public; again, not applicable here since the more appropriate way to protect the public from a doctor who is deemed to be a clinical danger is to stop him or her practising. Furthermore, by reinforcing the blame culture, this sentence is likely to increase the risk to other patients. Third, the punishment is intended to provide some kind of restitution to those who have been wronged. This may be an important consideration, but if it were the main factor determining how our criminal-justice system operates, we would still use the death sentence.

Perhaps the determining consideration is whether this punishment was just? I can only leave that judgement to the reader.

6 Testing times

Suck it and see

'It's all a bit disappointing,' Mo said, passing Daniel's charts across to Sebastian. 'His lung function is still going off. His FEV_1[1] is down to 65 per cent.'

It was the end of a long afternoon, and Daniel was the last patient to be seen. Susan had requested this slot particularly, so that they would have time to get back from his piano exam, which had fallen on the same day as the shared-care clinic at St Michael's.

Mo Khan, Daniel's consultant at St Michael's, had been running the shared-care clinic with Sebastian Hill for the past five years; in fact, ever since Sebastian had been appointed as consultant at the Albion. For children having 'shared care' between specialist and local hospitals, it was an ideal way for the consultants from both centres to work together. Several of the other hospitals in the area had such clinics for quite a while longer, and Val Sharpe had promised Mo that they'd get one established at St Michael's as soon as she managed to get another consultant in post to help with her massive workload. Mo knew Val was overstretched and grudgingly accepted her rationale for leaving him until last because he was more experienced in respiratory paediatrics than many of his district general colleagues. Nonetheless, he was very pleased when Sebastian was appointed, because it meant that families like the Johnsons only had to traipse up to the Albion for an annual review, and could otherwise be managed locally. And it was a good way for him to stay on top of the latest developments.

---

1 Test used to monitor lung function, and show if the lungs are being damaged. The figure is a percentage of what would be expected for a normal child of same age, so a falling FEV_1 is a bad sign.

Susan had been pleased too. As it happened, they had been on the ward at the Albion on the day that a barely recognisable Sebastian had appeared in his interview suit to tell the ward staff that he'd just been offered the job. Susan had only seen him intermittently over the intervening years, so she was a bit shy about breaking in on the teasing about Sebastian's formal attire. But she had eventually slipped over to shake his hand and congratulate him. Now, five years later, she felt very confident in the way the teams worked across the Albion and St Michael's.

'Think we'd better get them in and talk about a trial of azithromycin,' Sebastian said. 'How do you think this is going to go down? Susan seemed pretty flat last time we saw them six months ago.'

'Well, she's been up and down. I had a long chat with her when she was up here a couple of months ago. There are lots of other problems at home at the moment, and it's been very hard for her. Her daughter – Sara – moved in with her boyfriend a couple of months back, and three weeks later they both got picked up on some minor drug charge. Susan always thought the boyfriend was a liability but, predictably, the more she tried to talk Sara out of seeing him, the more she stuck her heels in. I also have a hunch that the marriage might be a bit rocky. Daniel's dad used to be the one who brought him for appointments, because he was working nights, but I haven't seen him for a few months, and Susan's made a few oblique comments about him.'

'Oh dear. It doesn't sound good. I think we're going to have to tread carefully,' Sebastian said. 'I'll go and call them in.'

'How's his FEV_1 then?' Susan asked as soon as they'd got through the opening pleasantries. 'Has it improved at all?'

'Not really, I'm afraid,' Mo said. 'In fact, it's down a wee bit.'

Susan had anticipated this response. She wondered how to phrase the next question. She needed to find out how serious the deterioration was without alarming Daniel.

'So how much has it gone down, then?' Daniel chipped in.

'About 6 or 7 per cent. Not too much, but we'd like to see it going the other way Daniel,' Mo said.

'Well, I am doing my physio properly.' Dan looked to Susan for confirmation. 'So this Tobi drug can't be doing much.'

'Fair comment,' Mo acknowledged. At just turned eleven, Daniel was bright and direct, and Mo knew that Susan's efforts to shield him from the implications of his illness were doomed to failure.

Mo thought back ruefully to the hours he'd spent on the phone six months ago, trying to get someone to take responsibility for funding Daniel's Tobi treatment. Daniel now had chronic *Pseudomonas* infection,[1] and at first had done well on regular colomycin, an antibiotic given through an inhaled mist. But, as is often the case, he had started to show signs of gradual lung damage, and Mo and Sebastian had decided to try him on Tobi, another inhaled antibiotic that was proving better than colomycin at arresting and even reversing this deterioration in a few patients. An easy decision clinically and a nightmare to put into practice – because at 1,500 pounds for a month's supply of Tobi, there was always a fight about who would pick up the bill. After the usual round of calls to Jack Stebbing, the PCT, his own service manager at St Michael's, the chief pharmacist at the Albion, Sebastian and back to the PCT, a deal had finally been agreed. St Michael's would pay for the first six months, and the PCT would pick up the bill after that if the drug proved its worth. So after telling his own service manager how crucial this drug was to Daniel's well-being, he was glad she wasn't here to hear it dismissed as 'not doing much' by an astute eleven-year-old.

'It's OK love, Dr Khan knows you're doing your physio,' Susan said. Trying to regain control from her son, she asked, 'So what's the next step?'

Sebastian joined in at this stage. 'There is another drug we'd like to try. It's called azithromycin, and it's showing some really promising results in reversing lung damage in children with cystic fibrosis.'

'You said that when we started the Tobi. So is there any way to know if this one will be any more effective?' Despite her resolve not to worry Daniel, she needed to ask the question, and she was rapidly accepting the fact that if she didn't, he would.

'Well, obviously there are no guarantees,' Sebastian said. 'But we've been very impressed with the trials that have been done with this drug. In fact, so much so, that we're starting to use it before Tobi these days.'

'So it's still an experimental drug then? Am I gonna be a guinea pig?' Daniel asked.

'No, no – not as such. It's actually been on the market since about 1991. The thing that's new is how effective it's turning out to be for cystic fibrosis. There was a very good study done recently that showed that about a third of children on this drug have an improvement in their FEV_1 of more than 13 per cent over six months.[2] And it also cuts the number of courses of additional antibiotics that are needed for acute infections. We don't fully understand how it works yet, but that's one for us to puzzle about.'

1 See Chapter 5
2 Equi et al. 2002: 978.

'The other good thing is that Daniel can take it by mouth,' Dr Khan said. 'And we won't have all the delays that we had starting the Tobi, because it's not such an expensive drug.'

Susan and Daniel were both well versed in processing information about FEV_1s, drug trials and the like. 'So if it does work, how long will Daniel be on it?' Susan asked.

'What we're doing at the moment is giving it every day for the first six months. Then, if there is an improvement, we're giving it three times a week after that.'

'But if it works, why not carry on having it every day?' Daniel asked.

Mo and Sebastian exchanged glances, and Sebastian replied to this question. 'The thing is Daniel, we're having to find our way a bit as we go along on this. We're breaking new ground, so we're not completely sure about the best long-term dose to give. This is our best hunch, based on the trials that have been done and our clinical instincts. We'd aim to keep a really close eye on things, and judge how we're doing by how your lung-function tests go. And, of course, we'll keep talking to you and your mum about the next steps at each stage.'

'I get it. So I would be a bit of a guinea pig after all. Sounds like we just have to suck it and see.'

Daniel dealt with the world with the black-and-white pragmatism of an eleven-year-old, but Susan still needed a bit more detail and reassurance.

'So we don't know if there are any long-term risks from children being on this drug for several years?'

'Well that's true, although it seems to be a very safe drug when used for other conditions. For example, lots of people take it for pneumonia and ear infections and so on. And we'll be monitoring things very closely. As you know, the most important thing now is to look after Daniel's lung function. That's our No. 1 priority. Set against that, we don't have any reason to suspect there will be any long-term adverse effects from the drug. As you know, we can never say never, but I'd be really surprised if it turned out to have any worrying long-term side effects.'

'And what about more immediate side effects?'

'In theory, the same as most of the drugs we use: nausea, diarrhoea, headaches, rashes and the like. But none of my patients have complained of any of those things. The other thing to watch out for is any effect on his hearing – and we also have to do some occasional blood tests to make sure it's not having an adverse effect on his liver. But really, Susan, it's proving to be a very well-tolerated drug, and we haven't had to take anyone off it that I've been seeing, either here or at the Albion.'

The uncertainty factor

'But how do we know it's not the azithromycin, Dr Khan?' Susan asked, indicating the letter from the school doctor that lay on the desk between them. Four months into his azithromycin treatment, Daniel's routine school hearing check had revealed a minor hearing loss. Susan had managed to arrange a quick chat with Dr Khan at the end of his morning clinic, while Daniel was still at school. 'I can't believe we could be this unlucky. Just when his FEV_1 has picked up by 10 per cent. We can't afford to stop his azithromycin now, just when he's doing so well.'

'Really Susan, let's not jump the gun. It's very unlikely to be related,' Mo said. 'The first thing we need to do is repeat the test. Most times when you get an abnormal hearing test in a child on azithromycin, it turns out to be normal when it's repeated. But if it's still down we'll get him seen in the Audiology Department. They'll be able to do much more detailed tests to work out exactly what kind of hearing loss it is. Then we'll have more idea of whether it could be drug-related.'

'I'm sorry, Dr Khan. I must drive you mad worrying about every possible worst-case scenario. You see, it's the uncertainty that gets to me. This azithromycin is just another example of how much of a gamble it all is. Even if this hearing problem isn't related, and he doesn't have any other side effects, without any really long-term studies we don't know if he'd do better on a higher dose or a lower dose, or taking it every day, or what. And if we take the wrong gamble, we can't go back and do it differently. He only gets one chance.'

Susan didn't pause for long enough to let Mo respond. 'Then, of course, there's the Internet. When you've got a child with an incurable condition, it's very hard not to keep surfing around, looking for the new drugs and the new cure that might be around the corner. Most of the time I just get on with things in a perfectly rational way, and then something sparks me off and I start reading all this stuff on the web, and wondering if one of these new treatments isn't the one that could help him. Sometimes I even think maybe I should take him off to Lourdes or something. That really makes Matthew angry, so I try not to talk about it.'

Mo realised that what he was hearing was the tip of the iceberg, and there were a huge number of worries bubbling under the surface for Susan. He thought he should really ask a few open questions that might encourage her to expand a bit more, but he had slotted her into a non-existent clinic space and he needed to get up to the ward to do a round with the new registrar, so he opted for trying to be reassuring. 'I think maybe people just have different ways of dealing with things, Susan,' Mo said. 'You go through flurries of surfing around looking for cures, and maybe Matthew tries to block it out more and not think too much about the implications. But what you're doing isn't irrational. Lots of people think about the miracles, and the things that are "on the edge" scientifically, because that's what gives them some hope for the future. As long as conventional medicine doesn't have all the answers, people will always look elsewhere. But, equally, some of the stuff you find on the Web is perfectly scientifically grounded, and Sebastian and I will always be happy to talk to you about new treatments that you've found, and tell you if there is good evidence for trying them.'

'Thanks Dr Khan. I really do appreciate that. I know you're busy, so I'd better stop rambling and let you get on.'

She stopped as she reached the door. 'But, you know what? In a way, I think Daniel copes better with this than either me or Matthew. He's always lived this way. On the one hand, the uncertainty about his treatment and, on the other hand, the certainty that he's never going to grow old. And he seems to accept it in a way that I just can't. Sometimes – even eleven years on – I still get angry about how unfair it is.'

'Anyway, I'm sorry Dr Khan. I think you just have me on a bad day. Honestly, I'm fine most of the time, but you know what makes it worse? It's the transitions. When Sara moved in with her boyfriend a few weeks ago, it wasn't the worry about Jake and the low-lifes he hangs round with that got to me most. It was thinking that maybe Daniel will never get the chance to set up home with a girlfriend. You see, he started his new school this term, and I went to the first open day last week. And I couldn't help thinking that maybe he won't be leaving with the other children. But then, I can't keep mourning for him at every celebration, can I?'

There was no time for Mo to reply, or maybe Susan didn't want him to, because she had vanished before he even had a chance to say goodbye.

Cut! Rewind

What do we want from our clinicians? Skill and competence is obviously crucial, but we also want respect and shared decision-making about treatment options. We would like them to know the answers – to be certain about the facts – because how else can we use those facts to make informed treatment choices? If we went to buy a car, we would expect the salesperson to be able to tell us something about the acceleration time from 0–60 m.p.h., the braking system, the petrol consumption, and so on; then we might decide that we would be prepared to trade off higher petrol consumption for better performance. Supposing the sales person didn't know? Supposing they said that the car hadn't been fully road-tested yet? We'd rapidly decide to look elsewhere – and it would undermine our confidence in that make of car and in the car dealership. Deciding on treatment options is much more important than buying a car. So how certain is the information that we're working with? How certain are the nurses, doctors, physiotherapists, pharmacists and others that the information they give us is accurate?

Susan found uncertainty difficult to deal with, as do we all. She wanted the answers to be black and white and the choices to be straightforward. Instead, she had to make decisions for her son that might turn out to be the wrong ones – and that was hard to bear. The decision to try Daniel on azithromycin was more straightforward than some, because both Mo Khan and Sebastian Hill were clear that this was the right thing to do and were able to give consistent advice based on sound research. But they were less clear about the longer-term treatment regime: whether it would be effective, whether the dose they were using was the best and whether there would be any long-term side effects. Making a decision about a treatment that has, for example, a 50 per cent chance of cure, a 15 per cent chance of minor complications and a 3 per cent chance of serious or long-term complications would be tough enough. What about making a decision when some of that data is unknown? When there is no information about long-term complications? Mo and Sebastian could make educated guesses, based on prior experience of similar drugs, but they couldn't give Susan proven risk data. Clinicians need to be able to share information with patients in a way that allows them to make decisions based on a full understanding of the facts. This can be particularly difficult when there is incomplete data or uncertainty about risk. In this chapter I will start to explore some approaches to this problem.

A closely related problem is that in a system that is resource limited, there is a pressure to prove that treatments are effective in order to justify funding them. The more expensive the treatment, the greater the burden of responsibility to prove that it works. But proving effectiveness is not enough. The fact that demand outstrips supply means that rationing must take place, whether explicitly or implicitly. Who should make the choices about whether to fund a very expensive treatment for a few individuals, when this might have implications for funding more routine treatments for many others? I will discuss some of the conflicts implicit in managing a health-care system in which resources are limited, whilst at the same time trying to preserve patients' rights to choice and treatment.

THE HEALTH-CARE SYSTEM: EVIDENCE-BASED CARE

'Give your evidence,' said the King; 'and don't be nervous, or I'll have you executed on the spot.' This did not seem to encourage the witness at all: he kept shifting from one foot to the other, looking uneasily at the Queen, and in his confusion he bit a large piece out of his teacup instead of the bread and butter.

(Lewis Carroll, *Alice's Adventures in Wonderland*)

Thus far, our discussions about the health-care system have focused on some of the operational practicalities of ensuring that such a large and complex machine works smoothly: practicalities such as staffing, communication, safety measures and structural organisation. It is equally important to understand the systems that are used to ensure that the care we offer and receive is the right care. How do we know that the treatments are effective and the best available? That the diagnostic tests are valid? That the predictions about illness and risk are accurate?

In Chapter 2 I began to explore some of the different cultural belief systems on which we base our understanding of illness and its treatment. We described how, in Western society, medicine is based on scientific rationality, a belief system in which all assumptions and hypotheses must be capable of being tested and verified under objective, empirical and controlled conditions (Helman 2003).

Of course, scientific rationality has not always been the dominant belief system. It had to fight for supremacy against the strongly held beliefs of the Catholic Church. In the early 1600s, the scientific method was to theorise about how things ought to work and to harmonise that thinking with the doctrines of the Church. Galileo Galilei challenged that method, basing his conclusions instead on experimentation and observation, an entirely novel approach that nearly cost him his life when his experiments led him to proclaim that the earth was not flat, but round. Galileo was imprisoned, but spared the death penalty, whilst the less fortunate Giordano Bruno, who did not have such influential friends to protect him, was burnt at the stake for advancing the heretical belief that the earth was not the centre of the universe. Only in 1992 did the Catholic Church exonerate Galileo and admit that their findings had been wrong.

At around the same time that Giordano Bruno met his untimely death, the British Royal Navy was struggling with a major threat to its global supremacy: scurvy. As early as 1594 Sir Richard Hawkins had recommended the use of 'sour oranges and lemons' to prevent the problem, but over a century later this treatment remained unproven, and far more men were dying of scurvy than were dying in action. James Lind, the man credited with being the 'Father of Naval Medicine', entered the navy in 1739 as a surgeon's mate (Jenkins 2004: 3). He was twenty-three years old, the same age at which today's medical students graduate as doctors. Lind was aware of the reported benefits of fruit and vegetables in treating scurvy and of the unsubstantiated nature of these claims. In 1747, he set up what was to be the first published 'randomised, prospective controlled trial' – one of the most important tools for assessing the effectiveness of medical treatments, and as relevant today as it was in 1747.

> Their cases were as similar as I could have them. They all in general had putrid gums, the spots and lassitude, with weakness of their knees. They lay together in one place, being a proper apartment for the sick in the forehold, and had one diet common to all.
>
> (Jenkins 2004: 3–4)

Lind chose twelve men with scurvy on HMS *Salisbury*, and matched them up in six pairs. He randomly allocated each pair to a different treatment. By just one week later the pair taking oranges and lemons were dramatically improved, whilst their shipmates on other regimes such as cider, seawater and vinegar were unchanged. Despite publishing his findings in 1753, it was not until 1795, a year after Lind's death, that the Admiralty finally took note of his recommendations and introduced lemon juice into the diet of all sailors, thus effecting a dramatic change in the health of the fleet, and in the course of European and world history.

Proving that treatments work

If Sir Richard Hawkins suggested a method for preventing and curing scurvy in 1594, how did it take 201 years to find its way into naval policy? Even allowing for the lack of seventeenth-century Internet cafés, this seems like remarkably slow progress. Certainly dissemination and adoption of new information was a factor, and an issue we will return to. However, a very important issue was the lack of a conclusive method for proving that the 'oranges and lemons' treatment worked at all, or that it was better than any other method. This was what made Lind's work so ground-breaking.

What is a randomised controlled trial?

A randomised controlled trial (RCT) is a study in which people are allocated at random to receive one of two or more clinical interventions. The aim is to compare the outcomes of the interventions – so a key feature is that the outcomes must be measurable. The interventions do not have to be drug treatments. They can be different kinds of speech therapy, acupuncture compared to drug treatment, or drug treatment compared to surgery.

It is very important that people are allocated randomly, as in Lind's example above. For example, if a new treatment is only given to the sickest patients, after all other treatments have failed, it is harder to show that it has an effect. Lind realised that his groups had to be as similar as possible, so that he could make valid comparisons between them.

RCTs often aim to compare the 'standard' or accepted treatment with a new treatment and, in this case, the people who receive the standard treatment are called the 'control' group. Another way of having a control group is for one group to have the 'active' treatment and the other group to have a 'placebo'. A placebo is a dummy treatment – for example, sugar-containing pills that look the same as the real drug.

This brings in another important feature of RCTs, known as blinding. If patients are put on a treatment that they believe will work – maybe a new drug – then they may well show a genuine improvement. In fact, they can even show a measurable improvement if put on a placebo, which shows just how important the mind, as well as the body is to the healing process.

Finally, there have to be enough patients in a study for the results to be 'statistically significant', because in a very small study a particular result could occur as a matter of chance. As the numbers in the sample get larger, it becomes less and less likely that a result was a chance happening, but it takes extremely large numbers to reduce the 'chance' element to practically zero.

Practical problems in conducting clinical trials

The advent of RCTs makes it sound as if certainty should be easy – as if all treatments should be amenable to testing, with clear answers about the risks and benefits. Unfortunately, this is far from the truth. There are many reasons why RCTs are not always practical or reliable, and a few are listed below:

Box 6.1 Learning points for clinicians and patients: some of the practical problems in conducting randomised controlled trials

- Sometimes it is not possible to make the groups similar enough; for example, patients in each group may be in the same age range and have the same disease pattern, but may turn out to be different in some way that is important to outcome – perhaps a difference in the sex ratio or racial mix.
- Sometimes it is not possible to recruit enough patients into the study to make the figures statistically significant. This is a particular problem if the study is evaluating treatment for a rare disorder, and in this situation many hospitals have to join in on the study to make it statistically viable.
- Studies can start with properly matched groups, but end up biased because more patients drop out from one or other group. This is important, because they could be dropping out because of a troublesome side effect, or because a treatment is not working.
- If the researcher is not 'blinded' and knows which group patients belong to, he or she may inadvertently treat or assess them differently. For example, if the researcher thinks that one treatment is better than the other, he or she may unintentionally exaggerate any positive reports about the treatment from patients in that group and minimise reports of side effects.

---

continued

- Some outcomes are easy to measure objectively, but others are very difficut; for example, response to a drug designed to reduce blood sugar is easy to measure numerically, whereas response to psychotherapy is more difficult to assess, because the measures are more difficult to design.

Ethical problems in conducting clinical trials

In addition to all the practical problems outlined above, there are many ethical problems involved in conducting clinical trials. In 1964, the World Medical Association developed the Declaration of Helsinki, which is a statement of the ethical principles governing clinical research. There have since been modifications to the declaration, as well as individual variations across different countries. However, one consistent outcome is that every clinical trial now has to be approved by a research ethics committee. Nonetheless, there are still many unresolved and difficult issues facing those involved in clinical research – both as investigators and as patients.

A particularly vexing problem is the issue of 'equipoise'. Equipoise refers to the situation where there is a genuine uncertainty about the relative merits of the treatments being evaluated. When this is the case, the ethical case for a treatment trial is relatively clear. On the other hand, if a doctor is certain that one treatment is better than another, then the traditional view has been that it would be unethical for them to enter a patient for a trial. In this situation, the doctor is ethically obliged to offer the treatment they believe to be best, regardless of whether that belief is based on a hunch or on solid evidence. However, in reality, doctors are often motivated to take part in trials precisely because they believe that a particular treatment offers better outcomes, so equipoise may be difficult to achieve. Benjamin Freedman has proposed an alternative view: that provided the medical community as a whole is uncertain about the relative merits of the two treatments (i.e. there is clinical rather than individual equipoise), then it is morally acceptable for a doctor to enter patients into a trial, regardless of their personal belief about the treatments (Freedman 1987: 141).

Not all clinicians would agree with this view, and many doctors would feel an absolute obligation to give their patient a treatment if they sincerely and wholeheartedly believed it was in their best interests. This means that responsibility for the welfare of the individual may well take precedence over the 'greater good' of resolving general uncertainty through a clinical trial (Weijer et al. 2000: 756).

However, there is a salutary commentary by Bill Silverman (2003), an American paediatrician who felt compelled, reluctantly, to conduct an RCT on a treatment that he had passionately believed was saving premature infants from blindness. The RCT revealed that the treatment was having no effect on visual outcome, but was exposing the babies to greater risk of life-threatening infections.

Clearly, informed consent needs to be obtained from all patients taking part in research trials. This is a much more complex and challenging task than obtaining consent in routine clinical practice (discussed further in Chapter 7), and it is important to be aware of two key differences: first, the benefits of the research may be uncertain and may not be experienced by the person participating in the research; second, the risk involved for research participants may be difficult to identify or to assess in advance and there may be unforeseen risks.

Researchers sometimes have to face extraordinary dilemmas in balancing ethics, risks and progress. For example, a group of clinicians who were conducting research into the management of HIV sought the help of a professional moral philosopher when confronted with the following problem (Tännsjö 1999: 449). They were conducting research on a new drug that they hoped would delay the transition from HIV infection to full-blown AIDS. They had some indication that the drug might be helpful, but this was far from conclusive and, meanwhile, data was emerging that showed that one in 500 patients was killed by the drug. Was it right to continue a trial of a drug that risked patients' lives and was not yet proven to confer any benefit? Or should they continue with the trial and allow individual patients to make their own decisions about entry, after being informed about the risks? Following extensive discussion, the majority view was that they should continue. This put the dissenting clinicians in an even more difficult position, because if they did not enter their own patients for the trial, the remaining patients would be risking their lives for a trial that might not yield conclusive results because of the smaller numbers.

Further problems beset both researchers and patients when experimental drugs for life-threatening conditions are only available within the confines of a clinical trial. One could argue that if a drug is being tested, surely patients should be able to try it, without having to join a trial. If it is their wish to try that drug, they are effectively being

coerced to join a the trial if that is their only means of obtaining it –
and even then, they risk being randomised to a different treatment
arm. If one is trying to safeguard the 'greater good', the counter-
argument would be that it is not right to allow patients to take
unproven treatments in this way, because this makes it impossible to
recruit enough patients for clinical trials and so gather the evidence
to find out if the treatment is truly effective. From a 'paternalistic' perspective, there is also the question of whether it is reasonable to allow
patients to take unproven risks with their lives.

Fortunately, in most trials, the decisions are not as difficult, and the
stakes not as high as this. Nonetheless, for any proposed trial, patients
need to have detailed information, presented in a form they can
understand, and adequate time to make a decision about taking part.
The following is a list of the topics that should be covered in a patient-
information leaflet about a clinical trial:

**Box 6.2 Learning points for clinicians and patients:
issues that should be covered in a patient
information leaflet about a clinical trial**

- The aims of the study and the question it is addressing.
- Alternative clinical options if the patient decides not to participate in the study.
- The demands placed on participants during the study,
  including laboratory and study testing needed for the
  research (and the risks of such testing).
- Known risks of the proposed treatment and the fact that
  there may also be unforeseen risks.
- The fact that participants may not benefit from participation
  in the study.
- Who to contact with scientific or ethical questions about the
  study – for example, the principal investigator or specific
  members of the research team.
- How personal data will be protected during and after the
  study.
- The fact that the patient can withdraw from the study at any
  time.

Clinical trials in children

The ethical problems involved in conducting research in consenting adults are great enough. The problems in children are even greater, and the same is true of other vulnerable groups – for example, those with a learning disability – who are not deemed competent to give informed consent. We need to conduct clinical research in children because we want them to be able to benefit from scientific advances. When compared to research on adults, many research questions relevant to the health of children have not been addressed at all, or only by small, poorly designed studies (Medical Research Council 2004). Unfortunately, because children are not small adults, only a limited amount of information can be extrapolated from the adult literature.

There are many reasons why research in children presents particular problems. First and foremost is the issue of consent. In paediatric research, consent is obtained by proxy from the child's parents. If children are old enough to understand, they should be involved as much as is possible in the process of decision-making. However, this still places a heavy burden on parents, particularly if there are risks involved. As in all research on patients, the emphasis is on minimising risk. Nonetheless, some degree of risk may be unavoidable, and parents inevitably find it harder to make this kind of decision on behalf of their child than for themselves.

Sometimes, the planned research is of no direct benefit to the child who is taking part, but is intended to benefit future children, so involvement is for altruistic reasons. This generally involves research other than clinical trials, such as collecting data on the progress of a disease or assessing methods for diagnosis or screening. In this instance, the parent who gives consent is being 'altruistic by proxy'. This is considered to be ethical, because of the intended benefits (Bush 2000: 370), but would become more questionable if the risk to the child went beyond minor discomfort (for example, taking blood tests). However, if a child becomes upset by a procedure, researchers must accept this as a valid refusal (Medical Research Council 2004).

There is a further reason for the paucity of research on children, particularly in relation to drug trials. This is not an issue of ethics, but of financial expediency. The problem lies in the 'licensing' of drugs for use in children. Most drugs that are used in the United Kingdom have a 'product licence'. To obtain this licence, the manufacturer has to submit information from clinical trials to the Government's Medicines Control Agency. The information should show that the drug works for the illnesses it claims to treat, that it does not have dangerous side effects, and that it has been made to high standards. The product licence will say whether the drug has been approved for use in children, and which medical conditions it can be used for. It will also give the approved dose and route of administration. For many drugs, it is not worth the drug company's while to carry out trials in children. This is because such trials are difficult and expensive, for all the reasons outlined above, and children often form only a small part of the potential market. As a result, it is estimated that between 50 and 90 per cent of drugs used in the paediatric population have never been specifically evaluated for use in that age group (European Commission 2004).

The Children's NSF (see Chapter 3) states that on children's wards around one-quarter of medicines are prescribed outside licensed indications ('off-label') and in general practice at least one in ten medicines prescribed for children are off-label or unlicensed. Parents will understandably be worried to be told that their child has been prescribed an unlicensed or off-label drug, although this will be safe for the vast majority of drugs used in this way. This is because paediatricians have so much experience of using drugs that have not specifically been tested in children and have a good understanding of the risks and benefits. Nonetheless, this is not a reason for drug companies to shirk their responsibility to remedy the situation. In the USA a 'carrot and stick' approach is being used to encourage drug companies to carry out drug trials in children (Sutcliffe 2003: 64). The carrot is a 'paediatric exclusivity provision' which grants the company an additional six months of patent protection if their product has been voluntarily tested on children. The stick is an absolute requirement to test products on children under certain specific circumstances (for example, if usage in children is likely to be high, or if there are likely to be risks associated with failure to license for children). European legislation is in progress to provide similar obligations and incentives to develop medicines for use in children, and this should be in place by 2006. Implementation will not be straightforward. It is likely to be difficult to maintain a balance between the ethical obligations to protect children from the dangers of inadequately tested drugs while also safeguarding them from the risks of clinical trials and preserving their right not to be passive participants in research activities that are not in their best interests.

Throughout this book I have emphasised the importance of good communication between health-care providers, but this is crucially important when prescribing new, unlicensed or off-label drugs. For children like Daniel, who is old enough to start taking some responsibility for his own treatment, it is particularly important to ensure that information about choices is presented in ways that he can understand, as well as his parents. This will be discussed in more detail later in this chapter, and in Chapter 7.

Box 6.3 Learning points for clinicians: guidelines on prescribing new, unlicensed or off-label drugs

- Legal responsibility for prescribing lies with the practitioner who signs the prescription.
- Communication between hospitals or with primary care needs to be timely, accurate and contain sufficient information about the medicine and diagnosis to enable another practitioner to prescribe. This should include an indication of duration of treatment, reasons for any changes and monitoring required.
- Many medicines are prescribed for uses outside their product licence (off-label or 'unlicensed') for a different indication or age group, or in a different formulation or dose. Where there is a substantial body of evidence to support the use of products in these ways, then a GP may be asked to prescribe, but they must be fully informed and must agree to the transfer of clinical responsibility.
- Shared-care guidelines can be useful to help such providers feel confident to accept responsibility.
- Prescribing responsibility should remain with the hospital if treatment is part of a clinical trial or where specialised monitoring is required.
- Patients participating in a clinical trial, their parents or guardians must be aware that there is no guarantee that the medicine will be continued at the end of the trial, irrespective of the results.
- Medicines should be approved by the Trust's Drugs and Therapeutics Committee before they are routinely used or recommended.

Research into practice

In the previous section, I focused on the issues involved in carrying out well-conducted treatment trials (or RCTs). However, medical knowledge and innovation is not just about the treatment of illness. There are equally important advances being made in developing tools for accurate and early diagnosis, in understanding causation and in screening and prevention.

When we consult a doctor, we expect them to be 'on top' of the latest information. I have already discussed the dilemma for Dr Stebbing, Daniel's GP, in keeping up with the huge breadth of information that he needed to help him care for patients ranging from eight days to eighty years of age. What does this mean in practice? Currently there are well over 10 million medical articles in press, and every month around 4,000 medical journals are published worldwide (Greenhalgh 2000), not to mention the plethora of information being released onto the Internet on a daily basis. The task appears to be impossible. Fortunately, help is at hand through several mechanisms, many of which have been touched on earlier in this book.

The discipline of evidence-based practice

It does happen exceptionally that a practising doctor makes a contribution to science; but it happens much oftener that he draws disastrous conclusions from his clinical experience because he has no conception of scientific method, and believes, like any rustic, that the handling of evidence and statistics needs no expertness.

(George Bernard Shaw, *The Doctor's Dilemma*)

The emphasis on the discipline of evidence-based practice has gained momentum over the past decade. Evidence-based practice is defined as 'the conscientious, explicit and judicious use of current best evidence in making decisions about the care of individual patients' (Sackett et al. 1996: 71). Put more simply, it is a more organised approach to helping clinicians ask the right clinical questions, to find the relevant papers, to appraise them in a critical and structured way and to decide if the findings can be applied to the patient sitting in front of them.

No matter what our job, we learn what we need to know by one of two methods: push- or pull-learning. In push-learning we are taught everything we might need to know, so that we can pluck the relevant information from our head when we need it. If we relied exclusively on push-learning, we would need to be alerted to every new paper in our speciality as it was published, so we could be ready in case we ever needed that information. Pull-learning is 'just in time' learning. We find there is something we need to know and, when that happens, we have to be confident that we can access the relevant information and apply it to the situation. Doctors' basic training is based on push-learning, and the same is true for most other disciplines, but a large part of their subsequent learning has to be 'pull-learning', and this is where evidence-based practice is such a powerful tool.

Some doctors look askance at the exponents of evidence-based practice and claim that they have always sought the most up-to-date information, read the latest scientific papers and based their decisions on 'best evidence'. Trisha Greenhalgh, a strong advocate for the discipline of evidence-based practice, does not believe this is true (Greenhalgh 2000). One major issue is that despite the mountain of medical research papers, very often the evidence just isn't there: only about one-fifth of medical interventions are based on any kind of sound scientific studies. In some cases, this is because it would be inappropriate and unethical to do a study on a treatment that is obviously life-saving – for example, a trial comparing the use of antibiotics with a placebo in the treatment of meningitis. The research literature is rendered even more incomplete by the well-known phenomenon of publication bias: journals are more likely to publish a study that shows positive results, when negative results are just as important. Other reasons for gaps in the evidence arise from the problems in conducting well-designed studies that have been outlined above.

As well as the gaps in the literature, there are two further problems. First, despite the fact that doctors and other clinicians have always read a wide range of scientific papers, they have not necessarily approached this task in a structured and critical way. Often, the busy clinician would skim an abstract, see that 70 per cent of patients had responded to a new treatment and fail to take note of the study design. If the study had been carried out on only ten patients, without a proper control group, and the sample was not representative of most people with that illness, there would be little point in even looking at the result section. The result is meaningless. The second problem is that a whole raft of other factors is more likely to influence clinicians than a well-conducted study, even one that they have critically appraised.

These include what the esteemed professor thinks is the right treatment, the doctor's own twenty-five years of personal experience or, perhaps more immediately, the patient they saw last week who didn't respond to a treatment and had a disastrous reaction, or perhaps did fantastically and unexpectedly well.

There are now measures and resources in place that favour a change in practice and behaviour. First, critical appraisal skills are being taught to all clinical professionals as a core competency, so that the upcoming generation will be better equipped to seek and assess relevant research findings. Second, there are now many sources of 'pre-digested' evidence including systematic reviews, critically appraised topics and professionally agreed guidelines. Finally, there is widespread Internet access in hospitals, GP surgeries and community-based practices, so that all clinicians should be able to run round-the-clock searches on the various medical databases, such as Medline and Cochrane. A list of a few relevant web-based resources is given below (also see Chapter 2):

Box 6.4 Learning points for clinicians: web-based resources

- PubMed, <http://www.ncbi.nlm.nih.gov/entrez/query.fcgi>. Key search site for medical literature, including clinical-query facility.
- National Electronic Library for Health, <http://www.nelh.nhs.uk>. Current health-care knowledge, designed for clinicians.
- The Cochrane Database, <http://www.cochrane.org>. Collection of critically appraised articles.
- Clinical Evidence, <http://www.clinicalevidence.com>. *BMJ* resource setting out best available evidence for a wide range of treatments.
- Centre for Evidence Based Medicine, Oxford, <http://www.cebm.net>.
- The James Lind Library, <http://www.jameslindlibrary.org>. Documents the evolution of tests of medical treatments.
- NHS Prescribing Support Unit, <http://www.psu.co.uk>.
- Discern, Decision-support <http://www.discern.org.uk>.

Learning communities

In October 2004, the *British Medical Journal* (*BMJ*) published a special issue that explored the question of whether evidence-based practice has made a difference – either to the behaviour of clinicians or, more importantly, to clinical care. There were both positive and negative views. One of the difficulties is that it is easier to study the impact on clinicians than the downstream outcomes for patients. Several of the articles were particularly helpful, because they highlighted commonalities in the way in which evidence-based practice appears to have an influence. The important ingredients were shared learning and distillation of views with other colleagues – and this needed to be in a clinical setting rather than a lecture theatre (Coomarasamy and Khan 2004: 1017, Gabbay and le May 2004: 1013, Horbar et al. 2004: 1004, Lockwood et al. 2004: 1020).

I discussed clinical networks in Chapter 3 as a means of breaking down organisational barriers and improving communication. Clinical networks have another purpose: they enable the development of learning communities. Not everyone can be a leader and innovator in every clinical area, so, by forming networks, usually involving a specialist or teaching hospital, best practice can be shared and disseminated rapidly and effectively. By working together, members of a clinical network can develop or adopt evidence-based guidelines on how to manage particular conditions, rather than everyone inventing the wheel in isolation. Sometimes the leader will be a researcher working in the specialist hospital. For example, in Daniel's situation, Sebastian Hill was based in the teaching hospital and, since he was involved in the latest cystic fibrosis drug trials, he was able to disseminate this information to Mo Khan and to the other local paediatricians. However, for some aspects of care, leadership may well come from a clinician working in the district general hospital or in the community.

All clinicians have a duty to stay up to date. Being part of a learning group or community is an important part of that process. Doctors have to produce evidence that they have attended relevant courses and conferences in order to be 'revalidated' (that is, to remain of the professional register). Changes in the NHS pay structure mean that other clinicians also have to demonstrate ongoing development in their knowledge and skills in order to move up the salary scale. Ensuring professional competence is a challenge: it means that everyone has to allow extra time to appraise and assess colleagues, but ultimately it is in the best interests of both patients and staff.

THE SOCIETAL CONTEXT: RATIONALISING OR RATIONING?

We have talked about how evidence is developed and how clinicians – individually and in groups – can take a rational approach to interpreting it. Evidence has its limitations and is only one piece of the jigsaw that clinicians and patients have to assemble to support decision-making – an issue I will return to later.

At the other end of the scale, while evidence is being used at a micro-level to inform care for individual patients, it is also being interpreted at a macro-level, to inform care for the whole population. The body responsible for this is the National Institute of Clinical Excellence (NICE). NICE was established in April 1999, largely in response to disquiet about 'postcode prescribing', the lottery by which the availability of drugs or other treatment differs across the country. It gives guidance on individual health technologies, the management of specific conditions and the safety and efficacy of diagnostic and therapeutic procedures. Its recommendations are based on best available evidence. Since January 2002, the NHS has been *obliged* to provide funding and resources for medicines and treatments recommended by NICE.

NICE's evaluations take into account not just the clinical effectiveness of treatments, but also the cost. A frequent scenario is that a particular treatment is shown to be better than the current standard treatment, but also more costly. Tobi, the drug that Daniel had tried before going on to azithromycin, is a case in point. Mo Khan had struggled to get payment agreed in order for Daniel to go on a trial of this drug, but around the country there is considerable variation as to whether treatment with Tobi is funded (*CF Today*, Summer 2004).

In situations such as these, NICE has to make a judgement about whether to recommend newer treatments. It makes that judgement based on the cost of additional 'Quality Adjusted Life Years' (or QALYs). A QALY is a notional measure that attempts to capture the quality, not just the quantity, of extra years conferred by a superior treatment. In this system, a year of perfect health would have a QALY value of 1, and anything less than perfect health would have a value of less than 1. This means that a treatment that gave two more years of perfect health would equate to 2 QALYs, but a treatment that gave three more years of rather poor health (rated, say, at 0.5) would only equate to 1.5 QALYs. Each treatment is judged on a case-by-case basis, so there is no absolute cut-off beyond which NICE would reject a treatment purely on grounds of cost-effectiveness. However, as an approximate guide, it would be unlikely to reject a technology with a ratio of 5,000–15,000 pounds per QALY and would need special reasons to accept technologies with ratios of 25,000 – 35,000 pounds per QALY or above.

In the year that NICE was launched, its chair, Michael Rawlins, said that there was 'no role for NICE in the rationing of treatments to NHS patients' (Rawlins 1999), a statement that was greeted with scepticism by Richard Smith, then editor of the *BMJ* (see Smith 2000). Rawlins has stuck to this assertion by divorcing considerations of cost-effectiveness and affordability (Rawlins and Culyer 2004: 224). Just because a treatment is cost-effective does not mean that it is easily affordable. Rawlins places responsibility for dealing with the fall-out of NICE's recommendations squarely on the shoulders of the Government, suggesting that if a recommendation proves to be unaffordable, it is up to the Department of Health and the Welsh Assembly Government to override NICE's guidance.

A thoughtful paper by Maynard et al. (2004: 227) raises a number of flaws in Rawlins's approach, and suggests some alternative strategies. Their starting point is that health-care rationing is inevitable and that it is inescapably the business of NICE to prioritise effectively. They question the ethical basis of weighting QALYs equally across the age range, regardless of who benefits and suggest the option of a 'fair-innings' approach, in which everybody is entitled to a 'normal' span of health. This means that more weight would be given to a treatment that gave three more years of life to a twenty-year-old than to a seventy-year-old. Clearly there is ethical merit in both sides of this argument. The paper also questions the topics chosen for evaluation by NICE, which have focused strongly on new technologies. As a result, there has been a rising cost to the NHS as new technologies are approved, without a matched focus on evaluating existing treatments that may be of no benefit and could be withdrawn. The authors propose that NICE should be given a notional or, better still, an actual, top sliced budget (that is, a centrally allocated allowance) to fund its recommendations. This would force it to examine the cost-effectiveness of existing treatments as well as new ones.

These proposals, while grounded in a pragmatic realism, might not be well received by the media, the pharmaceutical industry or the public. There has already been speculation about whether the Human Rights Act 1998, which came into force in October 2000, would provide a legal basis for individuals to challenge NHS decisions about resource allocation (Edwards 2004: 6). Prior to this, the best-known challenge to a Health Authority's decision about resource allocation was the case of Jaymee Bowen, known as Child B (Ham 1999: 1258).

Jaymee was a six-year-old girl whose plight came to the attention of the public in 1995, when she relapsed a few months after receiving a bone-marrow transplant for leukaemia. The paediatric leukaemia specialists looking after Jaymee felt that further treatment would have only a tiny chance of success and would expose her to further pain and discomfort. They recommended that it would be in Jaymee's best interests to offer her palliative care to make the last few weeks of her life as comfortable as possible. Jaymee's father was not willing to accept this advice and, with his daughter's life at stake, he sought further opinions. He received more optimistic advice about the possible success of more chemotherapy and a second transplant from doctors in the USA and adult leukaemia specialists in the United Kingdom. Mr Bowen asked Cambridge and Huntingdon Health Authority to fund this treatment. The Authority took the view that the paediatricians looking after Jaymee were best placed to assess treatment options and they were not prepared to use resources on an experimental treatment with limited chance of success. Mr Bowen sought a judicial review which resulted in the High Court asking the Health Authority to reconsider its decision. This judgement was subsequently overturned on appeal. Sir Thomas Bingham, then Master of the Rolls, said 'difficult and agonising decisions have to be made as to how a limited budget is best allocated to the maximum advantage of the maximum number of patients. This is not a judgement the court can make' (*R* v. *Cambridge Health Authority*, exp B [1995] 2 All ER 129, 133 (CA)).

Mr Bowen's fight to save the life of his daughter raises a number of important questions. The Health Authority was acting on the basis that high-cost treatment with a low chance of success was not justified. Their case was strengthened by the opinion of the clinicians that this might not even be in Jaymee's best interests since the harm might outweigh the benefits. The Health Authority pointed out that they had, at the same time as refusing to allocate an estimated £75,000 to Jaymee's treatment, paid out £200,000 for treatment for a patient with haemophilia. In the latter case, they were advised by the clinicians that the treatment was appropriate and effective.

Set against the Health Authority's responsibility to ensure effective and appropriate use of resources, there is a powerful drive to respond to the needs of an individual, particularly an individual whose life is at stake. The conclusion to Jaymee's story was that an anonymous donor provided the money for her to receive further treatment. This enabled her to survive for a few more months but, sadly, she died in May 1996. Would the public and media response to Jaymee's situation have been the same if she had been eighty years old rather than six?

One consideration is the 'fair-innings' rationale mentioned above. Jaymee had certainly not had a fair innings. But it is also hard to ignore the sanctity that is attached to the life of a child (see also Chapter 3, pp. 85–7), and that must have been close to the heart of the donor who so generously supported her treatment.

Three Articles under the Human Rights Act 1998, which has come into force since Jaymee's death, could be considered relevant to the issue of resource allocation. These are the 'right to life' (Article 2), the right not to be subjected to 'inhuman or degrading treatment' (Article 3) and the right to 'respect for private and family life' (Article 8) (see Chapter 3). Several cases have been brought, both in the United Kingdom and in Europe, that have cited violation of these rights as a justification for reversal of local health-care decisions. In every instance, the plaintiffs' cases have failed. The courts have held that rationing decisions are an inevitable consequence of the pace of medical advances, coupled with rising public expectation. However, the most important lessons that have emerged through all these cases have been that the decision-making process and priority-setting must be taken within a clearly defined framework that takes account of societal values, and is transparent and publicly accountable. This is summed up in a case in which three claimants challenged the decision of the Health Authority not to fund their gender-reassignment surgery. The Court of Appeal made the following points about the process of deciding on priorities:

> Although it is appropriate for a Health Authority to have a policy for establishing certain priorities in funding different treatments, in establishing priorities – comparing the respective needs of patients suffering from different illnesses and determining the respective strengths of their claims to treatment – it is vital for the Health Authority to:
>
> - accurately assess the nature and seriousness of each type of illness
> - determine the effectiveness of various forms of treatment for it, AND
> - give proper effect to that assessment and that determination in the formulation and individual application of its policy.
>
> (*North West Lancashire Health Authority* v. *A, D and G* [2000])

AT THE FRONT LINE: LIVING WITH RISK AND UNCERTAINTY

Medical knowledge is a vast commodity, which is expanding at an exponential rate. For much of the time we are dealing with well-established facts and well-understood treatments. But we have also learnt that medicine is an imperfect science and that sometimes we have to base decisions on a faulty and incomplete evidence base, and a mix of known and unknown risks and benefits. Regardless of the strength or weakness of the available information, doctors have a responsibility to present that information to patients in a way they can understand. Their next task is to help patients 'filter' the information through the lens of their own personal beliefs, priorities and preferences. The aim is to arrive at a plan that is specifically tailored for individual needs. In other words, 'off the peg' plans are generally a poor fit, and one size does not fit all.

Two skills are therefore required: the ability to communicate information and risk, and the ability to support decision-making. Perhaps not surprisingly, more attention has been given in the medical curriculum to teaching doctors how to communicate information than to communicate risk, so I will focus more specifically on the latter, and then move on to the issue of supporting decision-making.

Box 6.5 Learning points for clinicians and patients: the uncertainty factor

- Medicine is a science of uncertainties and probabilities.
- Scientific study can only shorten the odds, but cannot eliminate uncertainty.
- Where decisions have to be made in the face of uncertainty, clinicians and patients must do this in partnership.

Communicating information and risk

The importance of trust

> Trust is the key to communicating risk – as it is to so much. Lying
> destroys trust, but deluging patients with numbers doesn't build
> it. A risk is a combination of a probability of something hap-
> pening (where statisticians might be able to help you but often
> can't), a feeling of the dreadfulness of that event (which is very
> personal), and a context for the event.
>
> (Smith 2003: 0)

I have already discussed the important of trust in Chapter 3. John
Paling, Research Director of the Risk Communication Institute explains
that in communicating risk, trust is not an optional extra, but is an
essential prerequisite. Trust, as explained previously, is based on a
demonstration of competence and caring and, if this is not established
at the outset, the patient's risk perception will be skewed, regardless
of how clearly the facts are presented (Paling 2003: 745).

The importance of honesty

I have talked in Chapter 2 about the natural tendency of caring
professionals to resort to false reassurance. Nowhere is this more
dangerous than in the communication of risk. Everyone would like
medicine, airline travel and even walking down the street to be completely risk-free. Unfortunately, there is an irreducible risk associated
with all these actions. It is not possible to reassure patients that risk
is non-existent, but it is possible to reassure them that the risks of a
procedure have been identified and that safeguards are in place to
minimise those risks.

Communicating the numbers

Many doctors are confused by statistics (Smith 2003: 0), so it is
perhaps not surprising that they are poor at communicating them.
Two articles from a special issue of the *BMJ* (27 September 2003)

on communicating risk are particularly helpful in suggesting practical ways of communicating numbers more simply and effectively (Gigerenzer and Edwards 2003: 741, Paling 2003). Some of the key points from these papers are as follows:

Box 6.6 Learning points for clinicians and patients: communicating and understanding numbers

- **Wrong**: You have a 30 per cent chance of a sexual problem such as impotence on this drug. (Confusing for the patient – does this mean he could be impotent in 30 per cent of sexual encounters?)
  Right: 3 out of every 10 patients who take this drug has a sexual problem.
- **Wrong**: 1 in 25 people taking this drug get a rash, and one in 200 get severe headaches. (Some patients may think that a risk of 1 in 200 is bigger than 1 in 25.)
  Right: Use a common denominator: 40 in 1,000 people taking this drug get a rash and 5 in 1,000 get severe headaches.
- **Wrong**: You have a 3 per cent chance of dying on this treatment.
  Right: 97 out of 100 patients taking this treatment get better.
- **Wrong**: The probability that a woman has breast cancer is 0.8 per cent. If she has breast cancer, the probability that a mammogram will show a positive result is 90 per cent. If a woman does not have breast cancer, the probability of a positive result is 7 per cent. (What does this mean?)
  Right: Mammograms sometimes miss people with breast cancer and are sometimes positive in people who don't have breast cancer. 8 out of every 1,000 women have breast cancer. Of these 8 women, 7 will have a positive mammogram. Of the 922 women who don't have cancer, 70 will still have a positive mammogram.
- **Wrong**: If you have this treatment it will reduce your chance of dying by 80 per cent. (What does this mean?)

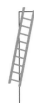

> **Right**: Out of 100 people with your condition who do not have this treatment, 5 will die, but out of 100 people who have this treatment, only 1 will die. If you have the treatment, you will be reducing the risk of dying by 4 in 100.
>
> (Gigerenzer and Edwards 2003, Paling 2003)

A picture is worth 1000 words, and visual information is a helpful adjunct to numerical data. John Paling's helpful article (Paling 2003), shows a number of visual tools that can be used.

Put risk in context and check understanding

Even with clear explanations of numbers, it is hard to put this in the context of everyday risk. Table 6.1 below, from the *BMJ* special issue, may be helpful. After imparting the facts, it is important for the clinician to try to check both the patient's understanding and response:

Table 6.1 Some familiar risks

Some familiar risks	Chance they will happen
Getting three balls in the UK national lottery	1 in 11
Dying on the road over fifty years of driving	1 in 85
Transmission of measles	1 in 100
Dying of any cause in the next year	1 in 100
Annual risk of death from smoking ten cigarettes per day	1 in 200
Getting four balls in the UK national lottery	1 in 206
Needing emergency treatment in the next year after being injured by a can, bottle or jar	1 in 1,000
Needing emergency treatment in the next year after being injured by a bed mattress or pillow	1 in 2,000
Death by an accident at home	1 in 7,100
Getting five balls in the UK national lottery	1 in 11,098
Death by an accident at work	1 in 40,000
Death playing soccer	1 in 50,000
Death by murder	1 in 100,000
Being hit in your home by a crashing aeroplane	1 in 250,000

continued

Table 6.1 continued

Some familiar risks	Chance they will happen
Death by rail accident	1 in 500,000
Drowning in the bath in the next year	1 in 685,000
Getting six balls in the UK national lottery	1 in 2,796,763
Being struck by lightning	1 in 10,000,000
Death from new variant Creutzfeldt-Jakob disease	1 in 10,000,000
Death from a nuclear-power accident	1 in 10,000,000

Source: *Electronic BMJ*, 27 September 2003. Reproduced with kind permission from BMJ Publishing Group.

Box 6.7 Learning points for clinicians: checking risk understanding and perception

Here are some examples of the kinds of questions that clinicians can use to check patients' understanding and response to the information given:

- Would you like me to run through those figures again?
- Is there any further information that you'd like about this treatment?
- Does that sound like a high risk to you?
- Would that put you off taking this drug?
- Is there anything I've said about this treatment that particularly worries you?

Collaborative decision-making

Armed with this information about how to communicate risk, is seems that Sebastian Hill and Mo Khan could have done better in their discussion with Susan and Daniel, and I will return to the issue of obtaining consent for treatment in Chapter 7. But they faced an additional problem, which was the uncertainty factor. They had a good RCT, which helped with the decision to put Daniel on a trial of azithromycin, but less evidence to support the longer term plans.

What are the important steps in helping patients to make an informed decision? There are four very different situations, each of which requires a different approach:

Box 6.8 Learning points for clinicians and patients: decision-making situations

1   **High benefit, low risk**: There is good evidence about the effectiveness, risks and benefits of the proposed treatment or intervention. There are very strong benefits, and the risks and side effects are minimal.

2   **Borderline risk-benefit**: There is good evidence about the effectiveness, risks and benefits of the proposed treatment or intervention. There are clear benefits, but there are also significant risks and side effects.

3   **Low benefit, high risk**: There is good evidence about the effectiveness, risks and benefits of the proposed treatment or intervention. There are only small benefits, but very significant risks and side effects.

4   **Uncertain risk-benefit**: There is not good evidence about the effectiveness, risks and benefits of the proposed treatment or intervention. There are reported, but unproven, benefits and unknown risks and side effects.

In order to be clear about which of these scenarios apply, the first step is to assess the strength of the evidence. RCTs are one source of evidence, but there are many lesser forms of evidence available. These include open trials (where there is no control or placebo group), case reports (reports of one of more patient responses) and expert opinion. It is beyond the scope of this book to cover this topic in detail, but a useful introduction can be obtained by visiting <http://www.cebm.net>. Professional readers are strongly urged to attend an evidence-based practice course.

Assessing the strength of the evidence is only one half of the equation. It is equally important to be sure that the results are applicable to the specific decision under discussion. A well-designed RCT of a drug that produced marvellous results in treating elderly patients with mild depression may not be applicable to a child who is severely depressed and suicidal.

High-benefit, low-risk situations

In many situations, there is strong evidence in favour of a particular treatment with minimal or non-existent side effects. Under these circumstances, it is usually easy to arrive at a decision and most patients would be happy to proceed. Nonetheless, it is important to remember that a side effect which may seem trivial to the doctor can be of great concern to the patient, and clinicians need to be sensitive to a wide range of preferences, as explained in the next section.

One important issue is that patients and clinicians may hold very different views about the categorisation of a decision. A high-profile example is the use of MMR vaccination, which has been the subject of media attention following claims that it is linked to the development of autism. Medical opinion is that MMR is safe and effective, and falls into Category 1 (high benefit, low risk), but many parents have taken the view that it falls into Category 2 or 3 and have opted not to vaccinate their children. The reasons for this marked disparity in risk perception are complex, but clearly loss of trust is one of a number of contributory factors. This is discussed further later in this chapter in 'At the end of the day'.

Borderline risk-benefit situations

In borderline risk-benefit situations, there can be very clear evidence about the positive and negative effects of the treatment, but it is a judgement call as to whether the benefits outweigh the risks or adverse effects. For example, women who have a very strong family history of breast cancer may be offered prophylactic mastectomy (that is, mastectomy as a preventative measure to avoid getting cancer). There is good evidence that this reduces their chances of getting cancer more effectively than screening and other prophylactic methods (Hartmann et al. 1999: 77), but it is clearly an extremely difficult and painful decision.

This highlights the most important point about decision-making in all but the most clear-cut situations: risk perception and risk-benefit ratio are things that are absolutely owned by the patient. They are a complex function of their experience, culture, values, beliefs and preferences. Some values are more obvious than others: for example, a procedure that carries a risk of slight facial scarring may be perfectly acceptable to a boxer, but wholly unacceptable to a model. However, there are much more subtle influences. Risk perception is altered by experience and some risks may be intolerable to particular individuals. These may operate at a conscious or unconscious level. Perhaps a relative suffered a similar complication. Perhaps a friend died of this illness. Perhaps a course of chemotherapy with severe side effects and minimal chance of reducing recurrence would be worthwhile, because regretting the missed opportunity would be unbearable later.

In these scenarios, there is no 'right' or 'wrong' decision, and the role of the clinician is to help the patient weigh up the available information to reach a conclusion. The most valuable resource for the patient is often time and the option to discuss the possibilities with friends or relatives as well as to revisit them with the clinician. Once a problem has been diagnosed, the patient will often feel under pressure to start on treatment. Clearly some treatments are urgent, but in many cases, a delay will be of no clinical importance at all. If this is the case, reassurance that there is no urgency to make the decision can be a huge relief, and taking away the pressure can make the decision-making process considerably easier.

Low-benefit, high-risk situations

This category includes chemotherapy in a patient who is already terminally ill, a major operation in a patient who is very frail and unwell, or surgery that has a high mortality or may leave a patient very disabled. Once again, judgements are highly personal.

As explained in relation to MMR vaccination, conflict between patients and clinicians can arise if there is a different perception about categorisation of a decision. For example, in the case of Jaymee Bowen, discussed earlier in this chapter, the doctors advised that further treatment fell into Category 3 (low benefit, high risk), but Jaymee's father assessed the treatment as being in Category 2 (borderline risk-benefit, and worth the risk).

Uncertain risk-benefit situations

Decision-making in the face of poor evidence and uncertainty is perhaps the most difficult scenario to tackle. In conditions where there are no effective or proven treatments, the dilemma is often made worse, because patients can be confronted with a confusing array of alternative therapies on the Internet. Sorting the wheat from the chaff is a daunting task. Autism is a good example of this problem. Many people will be familiar with the symptoms of autism, through the pop-ular film *Rainman* and through many documentaries on the television. The outcome for children with autism can be significantly improved by a range of educational and therapy approaches, but sadly there are no proven cures for the condition. Nonetheless, there have been a huge number of widely publicised claims of 'miracle cures' including injections of a drug called secretin, special diets, vitamin supplements, holding therapy (in which children are forcibly restrained until they stop resisting and give eye contact) and swimming with dolphins.

Regardless of whether a proposed treatment is a drug recommended by a doctor, a special diet identified by the patient, a physiotherapy technique or an educational approach, people have to find a way of deciding whether to embark on an approach that has uncertain risks and benefits. Just as importantly, once on the treatment, people need to have a way of deciding whether there are benefits that outweigh any disadvantages and side effects, and whether it is worth continuing.

The following questions might be helpful in making a decision to try a treatment or therapy approach:

Box 6.9 Learning points for patients: questions to ask before deciding to try a treatment with uncertain outcomes

- What positive results have been reported for this treatment?
- Has there been a scientific study, or are the positive reports all from individual patients?
- What side effects or risks have been reported for this treatment?
- What are the main symptoms that I hope will improve, and has the treatment been used for these particular symptoms?
- Has the treatment been used in people of my (or my child's) age, and with my (or my child's) symptoms?
- What will the impact be for the rest of the family (for example, financial costs, time costs and so on)?
- How easily can I get this treatment?
- How will I know if it has worked?

Some of these points can be explained further by following through on the example of autism. Autism affects different children in different ways, so that every child has a unique mix of abilities and problems. Some drugs have been shown to be effective in reducing the very troublesome obsessions that dominate the lives of many such children – but those who do not have problems in this area would not benefit from the same drugs. In other words, just because a treatment is effective for one subgroup of children with autism does not mean it would be useful for all children with this diagnosis. Specialist intensive educational approaches have been shown to improve attention and learning for some autistic children, but they require many hours of input on a one-to-one basis. The cost of this intervention (which is not readily funded by local education authorities) can be prohibitive for the family and can have consequences for the child's siblings. There are also reports that quite restrictive diets can improve outcomes for autistic children, but there is a risk of nutritional deficiencies on a restricted diet if it is not monitored very closely.

All these uncertainties means that patients and families need to make a careful balance sheet of pluses and minuses before deciding to embark on a treatment. Once that decision has been made, it is equally important to have a way of assessing whether the treatment has been useful. No one wants to continue a difficult, costly or inconvenient treatment indefinitely if it is not doing any good or, worse still, if it is proving harmful. Therefore the following advice is particularly important for treatments that are unproven, but applies *equally well* to treatments that are proven, but that work better in some individuals than in others:

Box 6.10 Learning points for patients: assessing the outcome of a treatment

- Decide on a 'target symptom' that is going to be used as an 'outcome measure'.
- Get a diary and start keeping a record of when the symptom occurs, so you can get a 'baseline' of how frequent it is before starting the treatment.
- Once the treatment has started, continue monitoring the target symptom in the diary.
- Set a deadline for reassessing the symptom. You need to take account of how long the reports say that the treatment takes before it starts to work.

---

continued

- Make a note in the diary of any side effects or problems.
- Once you reach the deadline, go through your results carefully (this may be with a doctor or another professional) and decide whether the frequency or severity of the symptom has improved enough to justify continuing with the treatment.
- Sometimes you may be looking for a feature that is improving or increasing rather than decreasing. For example, the time that a child with ADHD (hyperactivity and attention problems) can focus on a task before and after starting on drug treatment.
- Try to avoid starting on more than one treatment or changing more than one thing at once, because it will be difficult to decide which one is responsible for any benefits or problems.

Let's consider the example of a child with epilepsy who is starting on a new drug or a special diet. In this case the 'target symptom' is easy: the child's seizures. Picking the target symptom on a trial of evening primrose oil for premenstrual syndrome might be more difficult: it could be breast tenderness, bloating or moodiness, or a combination of all three.

It is very tempting to start something new right away without waiting to get a baseline or keeping a diary. The problem with this is that it is very easy to lose track of how bad things were at a point in time, as one busy week merges into the next, and the ups and downs of symptoms become a blur. The time taken to get a good baseline will vary depending on how often the target symptom occurs. For a child who has fits several times a week, a two-week diary would probably be long enough to get a good 'baseline' frequency.

It is also a good idea to have some idea of what sort of improvement you are aiming for. Will it be good enough to reduce the fits from three a week to one a month? Sometimes there has to be a compromise. For example, in the child with epilepsy, it may be that the dose of medicine to reduce the fits to once a month causes no side effects at all, but increasing the medicine enough to stop the fits completely makes the child unacceptably drowsy.

In all these situations, scientists can carry out research to look at outcomes for the population and for the majority of patients, but when it comes to assessing the outcome of the treatment for the individual, patients have be their own scientist and make their own personal decisions about the results of their treatment. It is hard to make these self-assessments completely conclusive because sometimes – despite best efforts to take a 'scientific' approach – other factors interfere: maybe a move to a different climate, a new therapist or a change in diet. Nonetheless, this kind of approach does give a degree of control and some guidance in decision-making.

At the end of the day

'You're even later than you said you'd be,' Yasmeen called from the sitting room, as Mo hung up his coat and glanced at the post on the hall table.

'Yes, sorry Yasmeen,' Mo replied. 'Afraid I got caught on the ward talking to some parents who couldn't decide whether to have a feeding tube put into their baby's stomach.' He stuck his head round the door. 'Did you eat with the children?' he asked.

'No, I waited. I had to survey a building in South London, so I had a late lunch. I've left ours ready to reheat in the microwave.' She followed him into the kitchen. As the microwave was whirring, she asked, 'So why was it such a difficult decision?'

'You mean the feeding tube?' Mo was interested that she had chosen to pursue this. 'Well, just think what it would have been like if we'd ever had to make that decision ourselves. The baby has real difficulty swallowing. It takes over an hour to give her each meal, and she's very underweight. But feeding your child is such a basic maternal instinct . . . it must feel so difficult and unnatural to end up doing that largely via a tube. Although actually you'd be surprised – once parents have made the leap and had the operation, they usually say they wish they'd done it sooner.'

'It must be terrible,' Yasmeen acknowledged. 'But still – couldn't someone else have spoken to them at this time of the evening – on a night when you're not even on call?'

'Probably. But they really wanted to talk to me, and they got held up in traffic on the way back to the hospital. Their baby has a very rare syndrome and I was the one who made the diagnosis after someone else missed it – so they tend to trust me more than any of the others.'

'There are some distinct disadvantages being married to every parent's favourite paediatrician. Too many lonely evenings and late dinners. Mind you, I was watching a programme on the telly before you came in, and I think you must be the only paediatrician in the country that everyone does trust.'

Mo took their food over the table and looked at her in surprise. 'What makes you say that? What was it about?' he asked.

'MMR and autism. I hadn't realised just how much the vaccination rate had fallen since that paper linking MMR and autism – and apparently measles infection has shot up. Anyway, they were talking about the furore that's erupted since it turned out that this chap Wakefield, the lead author, had a conflict of interests. You probably knew about it already, but I hadn't realised he was being paid by the solicitors of the families who were trying to sue the vaccine manufacturers. The most interesting thing, though, was the reaction of the public. They talked to a few parents who were due to have their children vaccinated and, although Wakefield seems to have been discredited, several of the parents still trusted him more than the Government or the paediatricians who say MMR is safe. So they said they weren't going to get their kids vaccinated.'

'That doesn't surprise me,' Mo replied. 'There's a big difference between how much parents trust me on a personal level, and how much people trust doctors in general – and government doctors or scientists in particular.'

'I suppose so. Maybe it's because paediatricians have been at the centre of so many of the high-profile scandals; there was the organ-retention business at Liverpool, then the Bristol heart babies, and then MMR and autism. Not to mention that paediatrician who testified against the mothers in those awful cot death cases.'

'It's certainly not a great catalogue of events,' Mo agreed. 'But I think it's more complicated than that. One big problem is that newspapers editors don't have to worry about improving the health of the nation. Their job is to sell papers, so they're always going to publish the more sensational stuff. Half the time, they've chosen which side of an argument they're going to support, and then it's like supporting one political party – they're always going to spin it from that perspective. Plus the media always hype up the risks of new scientific advances, and food scares and dangers to kids.'

'So you reckon it's all down to irresponsible reporting then?'

'Actually, no – I don't. There are two other really important things about this. First of all, the medical profession and the government have made some completely wrong assumptions about how the public respond to risk. It's daft to think that people base their reactions on some kind of data analysis. Of course they don't. People are much more sensitive to risks that have high consequences, like being killed in an earthquake or a plane crash, and they under-estimate some far more likely risks, like getting diabetes or heart disease.[1] Then, of course, the other thing that really jacks up anxiety is if they feel threatened by something they can't control – like mobile phone masts.'

'I suppose that's why I get in such a state about getting on a plane,' Yasmeen said. 'But surely there must be some way of getting messages across about what is and isn't safe?'

'I think quite a lot comes down to individual doctors. If a patient trusts their own doctor, or practice nurse, or whoever, they will have far more of an impact than the media campaigns. Particularly if different media sources are giving them contradictory messages. But the hard truth is that people don't base their decisions purely on what we say to them. They'll balance my view against other people they trust: their mother, their aunt, other mums they run into at the nursery. I'm not as influential as I'd like to think I am.'

'Quite right, you're not,' Yasmeen replied. 'Certainly not in this house. After everything you said to Taqi about choosing football rather than rugby at school, he's gone for rugby, because his best mate has chosen that. So I'm afraid you're going to have to live with the risk of contact sports.'

'Hmm. It's all very well my telling other parents that they have to let their children make their own decisions. It's a bit harder when it comes home to roost.'

'Welcome to the real world, Mo. But you said there were two important things?'

'Yes. The other one is uncertainty. Medicine just doesn't have all the answers, however much we wish it did. The whole business about Roy Meadow and the cot-death cases is very different from MMR. That wasn't about balancing probabilities for the greater good. It was about using an inexact science to help decide whether to send a woman to prison. Medicine is designed to help us counsel about risk and to support people in making decisions. It's not designed to make those kinds of judgements.'

'Of course it is, Mo. You can't cop out like that. Forensic scientists have been using medical science that way for decades.'

'OK, I suppose you're right,' Mo agreed reluctantly. 'But it wasn't the way I thought about using medicine when I decided to be a paediatrician.'

1 Mo had read about the public perception of risk in an article by Alaszewski and Horlick-Jones (2003).

UNRESOLVED QUESTIONS: FIRST, DO NO HARM

Uncertainty is not just the enemy of medicine. In science more broadly, in economics, in religion – indeed in every walk of life – the public is seeing an end to the authority that comes with certainty. On the one hand, a sharing of uncertainty is the only rational basis for a mature relationship between the public and its appointed leaders and scientists. On the other hand, it is hard to let go of the belief that 'experts' should be able to call on sophisticated tools and knowledge to provide sure and safe answers to complex questions. There is still an expectation of those vested with the mantle of authority and expertise and when they fail, the response is disappointment and, in some cases, anger.

Naomi Marks's article, 'An Expert Witness Falls from Grace' (Marks 2003: 110), describes the dramatic U-turn in the public perception of Sir Roy Meadow, Professor of Paediatrics and former president of the Royal College of Paediatrics and Child Health. Through 2003, Sally Clark and Angela Cannings, who had both been convicted of murdering their sons, had their convictions overturned by the Court of Appeal, whilst in a third case, Trupti Patel was found not guilty of murdering her three babies. Sir Roy, who had been widely regarded as a leading authority in the field of child abuse, had been a key prosecution witness in all three cases.

As each successive case hit the news-stands, Sir Roy was progressively demonised by the media and became the subject of increasingly vitriolic personal attacks by campaigners. Fitzpatrick (2004) described the febrile climate within which the debate developed as one marked by growing hostility towards scientific expertise in general and the medical profession in particular. Contemporaneous campaigns focused on issues such as animal experimentation, Gulf War Syndrome, genetically modified food and immunisation, all revealed a growing distrust of expert opinion.

It has subsequently been demonstrated that Roy Meadow made assertions that were not scientifically sound, and he has been struck off by the GMC after being found guilty of serious professional misconduct. However, this does not detract from the need to question whether it is the expert witness or the adversarial criminal-justice system that is ultimately responsible for conviction, with all its consequences.

Whatever the culpability in the cases that have now closed, the more sobering reality is the absolute inevitability that paediatricians will make errors in such cases in the future. They will do so because the art of medicine is just that – it is in large part an art, not a science, and hence fundamentally flawed as a means of providing irrefutable evidence in criminal proceedings. And for that reason its practitioners are condemned to do harm.

Despite popular belief, the Hippocratic Oath does not and never did contain the words 'First, do no harm'. However, the opening sentence of the Law of Hippocrates is perhaps more apposite.

> Medicine is of all the arts the most noble; but, owing to the ignorance of those who practice it, and of those who, inconsiderately, form a judgement of them, it is at present far behind all the other arts.
>
> (The Law of Hippocrates, circa 400 BC)

What do we know of the facts in these cases, and what can be done to minimise harm through misdiagnosis more generally?

In the first instance, we know that in a small number of cases parents and guardians can and do abuse, maim or kill their children. Apart from the all-too-familiar cases of systematic abuse such as Maria Colwell, Jasmine Beckford and, most recently, Victoria Climbié, a rather different psychological profile underlies the well-documented cases of parents who smother their infants. For example, one mother who murdered three of her children (Stanton and Simpson 2001: 454) formed an intense attachment to her first victim and described killing her because she was unable to bear her apnoea attacks[1] and her fear of losing her.

The second uncomfortable reality is that diagnosis, whether of child abuse or more conventionally testable medical conditions, is an uncertain business. Although in this chapter, we have focused on the uncertainties of treatment options, similar problems beset us in making diagnoses. But why should a diagnosis only have a 95 per cent or a 99 per cent chance of being correct? Surely you either have a disease or you don't?

It is true that there are some absolute realities: for example, pregnancy is an 'all or none' phenomenon; you can't be a little bit pregnant.

---

1 An episode where the baby stops breathing transiently, common in premature infants, and also a cause of cot death.

Fortunately, pregnancy tests are now very accurate in making the diagnosis at a very early stage. By contrast, screening for cervical cancer is not as accurate. There are both 'false positives' and 'false negatives'. What this means in practice is that because the stakes are so high (in that it's vital not to miss cases of cancer), it is important to set the threshold very low, and to call women back who have even remotely suspicious cells on their smear. So in order to 'catch' as many real cases as possible, a lot of perfectly healthy women have the worry of a smear recall. But most would accept that this is a safer, if stressful, option. The smears of the healthy women who get called back are called 'false positives'. Sadly, even by erring on the safe side, and by calling back a lot of healthy women, there will still be a few 'false negatives'; smears that seemed normal despite the fact that there were early cancer changes. The lower the threshold is set, and the more healthy women who are called back, the smaller the chance of false negatives (of missing early cancer changes). But that risk can never be zero. Earlier in the chapter (see p. 194) we gave a similar example for breast-cancer screening.

In child protection, a false positive has equally serious consequences, as the cases described above demonstrate. It can mean destruction of a family unit, catastrophic psychological consequences for the child and family, and even erroneous criminal conviction. And, for the paediatrician concerned, guilt, recrimination and public censure. But the false negatives can be equally frightening, as the following quote indicates:

> It is a chastening experience to perform a frank homicide necropsy[1] on a child whose elder sibling was signed off as a cot death a few years previously. I should know – I have done it.
>
> (Green and Limerick 1999: 697)

So where lies the greater harm? To risk the death of another child or the destruction of a family? A study by the Royal College of Paediatricians and Child Health found that 14 per cent of paediatricians had had an official complaint made against them in respect of child-protection issues, many of which had resulted in unpleasant local

---

1 Post mortem examination.

or national publicity, yet only a tiny proportion were upheld (Craft and Hall 2004: 1309). Prior to the recent judgement on Roy Meadow, of 87 paediatricians referred to the General Medical Council whose cases have been completed, none were found guilty of serious professional misconduct. It is perhaps not surprising that faced with this dilemma, paediatricians are running shy of child-protection work; 30 per cent of child-protection posts are unfilled.

A better way forward has to be found, in the interests of all concerned. Proposals for a non-adversarial approach to evaluating the evidence are commendable (Craft and Hall 2004), alongside plans for clearer procedures, and dedicated, skilled teams for investigating and managing sudden infant death. Nonetheless, the ongoing hostility and distrust that prevents constructive debate from taking place in an atmosphere of mutual respect must be laid to rest if children, families and professionals are going to be protected from harm. Medicine will always be an uncertain business, and ways have to be found to acknowledge this, while still retaining public trust.

7 Hard graft

Transplant decisions

Mother Teresa

'Are you going out of your way to kill yourself then?' Sara asked. When that produced no response, she continued, 'You're a bloody idiot. You know that, don't you?'

'Yeah, right. If you say so,' Daniel replied, keeping his gaze fixed firmly on the football match on the television.

'Dan, they're never going to give you this heart–lung transplant if they find out you're smoking and drinking like this. You're not a baby, you're fifteen years old. When are you going to grow up and take some responsibility for yourself?'

Daniel looked at Sara for the first time and, very deliberately, moved the empty beer can to one side and pulled the tab from another. Then he turned his back on her, picked up the remote control and turned the volume up to an uncomfortable level. Sara reached the end of her tolerance. She walked over to the socket on the wall and pulled the plug out.

'Hey, I was watching that!' Daniel shouted. 'Why don't you just butt out and mind your own business?'

'You weren't watching it, and you are my business. You're my brother, for God's sake, Dan. Does mum know you're smoking again?'

'No, of course not. Unless little Miss Snoop has run off and told her.' He glared at her in fury, trying to read whether she had or not. 'Like you're Mother bloody Teresa yourself. At least I haven't been picked up for doing drugs, like you were when you were with that creep Jake. So, just remind me, how many do you smoke a day now? Twenty is it? Of maybe you've gone up to thirty?'

'Look, that's not the point, Dan,' Sara said. 'I don't have cystic fibrosis.'

'No, that's right you don't – you picked the right father. So you don't have a clue what it's like. Don't you think I'm enough of a freak already?

What with this gastrostomy,[1] sticking out of my belly and not being able to stay out overnight because I need my pump feeds and my physio and my drugs and all the rest? And not being able to play football, or handle more than half a dance at a disco before I get out of breath? That's really going to help me pull a girl, isn't it?'

There was a momentary silence, and then he said, 'So why d'you suppose I'm here by myself on a Saturday night? It's because my mates have all gone off youth hostelling for the weekend.'

'OK, so maybe you can't go and climb the Three Peaks, or whatever it is they're doing. But you can stay out for the night. You just need to plan ahead a bit.'

'Plan ahead a bit?' Daniel replied. 'Sure. Just like you always did at my age. Look Sara, all the other blokes smoke. It's the only thing I can do that's anything like normal.'

'Oh great. So if all the other blokes went and jumped off a cliff, I suppose you'd just follow them?'

Daniel didn't respond for a moment. Then he said quietly, 'Yes, I think maybe I would. It would probably be a whole lot better than this.'

Sara looked at the clock. It was one in the morning, but she couldn't get off to sleep. Eventually she went back downstairs to make herself a cup of tea. It wasn't just Daniel on her mind. She was also worried about her mother. Matthew had left them three years ago and over the past couple of years, as Daniel's lung function had got remorselessly worse, Susan's whole life had revolved more and more tightly around her son. Sara sometimes felt guilty and wondered if she should have moved back home to help, but she knew couldn't face that. She was pleased that at least her mum had agreed to go and stay with friends in Ireland this weekend – her first break in ages – while Sara stayed in the house with Daniel.

Right now, Sara could have kicked herself. Somehow, Daniel always managed to get the better of her in these arguments. She was angry because he hit below the belt. When he threw his illness at her like that, she knew there was no real comeback. She couldn't be inside his body or his head. He was right: she didn't know what it was like. But there was one thing she did know. He had to have this heart–lung transplant. It was his only hope. He was due to go into the Albion the following week for a four-day admission to assess his suitability. Apparently there were some

---

1 Many children with cystic fibrosis have difficulty maintaining their weight, so they often have a gastrostomy – a feeding tube into the stomach – to help them get enough calories through extra liquid feeds.

medical tests and a whole series of meetings with nurses, doctors, psychologists and the like. Sara couldn't see how it was going to take four days of meetings. As far as she was concerned, this one was a no-brainer. Daniel had to have this transplant, or he would die.

Net benefits

'I just want to reassure you that we're not here to make a decision either way today. The main point of this meeting, and of the next few days, is to find out what you know already and to give you as much information as you need to help you make an informed choice.'

They were five minutes into their meeting with Emma Jay, the nurse specialist from the transplant team, and Sara was already starting to feel agitated. Her mother was fighting back tears, and Daniel was busy tracing a pattern with his finger on the sole of his trainer.

'Look, we've already made the decision,' Sara said. 'I've looked up loads of stuff about this on the net and printed it all out for Mum and Dan to read. We know all about it.' She pulled a sheaf of papers from her bag and put them on the table between them, just in case anyone needed any further convincing. 'There may be some families who take forever to make up their minds, but we just want to go ahead. I don't see why we have to waste all this time talking.'

'Sara, I don't think we do know enough about it,' Susan said, reaching for a hanky. 'There's so much information, and I haven't managed to read it all.'

'Mum, you don't have to read it all. The only question you have to consider is whether you want Dan to have a chance for a better quality of life or not.'

'I can understand why you are keen for your brother to go ahead with this,' Emma said. 'We just need a bit of time for everyone to go at their own pace, and to feel confident in their decision – most of all Daniel. So if it would help I'd be very happy to see any one of you individually.'

'Individually? What the point of that?' Sara said, her voice rising. 'I thought we were supposed to be making this decision as a family.'

Emma had been in this position many times. It was not unusual for one member of a family to dominate the discussion, making it hard to find out what the diffident adolescent in the midst of the situation really wanted. She looked at Daniel and said, 'Maybe it would help if you started by telling me what you know about the operation.'

Once again, it was Sara who answered. 'Sure. As I understand it this operation is Dan's only chance. If he doesn't have it quickly, things will only get worse. So the sooner we get on with it the better.'

'Sara, the important thing to understand about the timing is that even if Daniel does decide he wants to go ahead, it takes an average of twelve to eighteen months to get a transplant.'

'Twelve to eighteen months?' Susan said, looking stricken.

'Twelve to eighteen months on average.' Emma repeated. 'That means that some children get a transplant almost immediately, but I'm afraid that in some cases it's much longer – and unfortunately 50 per cent of the children who go on the waiting list never get a transplant.'

'Well that just proves my point,' Sara said. 'The sooner we get on with it and get his name down, the better. We have to think positive and have faith that he's going to be out there soon – playing football and enjoying life again.'

'Sara, I don't think it's that simple,' Susan said. 'It's a very big operation, isn't it?' She looked to Emma for confirmation.

'Yes, it is a big operation,' Emma said. 'Obviously if we find a suitable donor, and if the operation is successful, it could dramatically improve Daniel's quality of life. But it is important for him to understand that at the outset he will have to be on intensive care, on a ventilator . . .'

Daniel looked up and spoke for the first time. 'I've seen that kind of stuff on *Holby City*,' he said. 'It's like a blood bath. There are always people dying left, right and centre.'

'That's great. I hope you're pleased now,' Sara said to Emma. 'You've done a really good job of scaring Dan.' Then turning to Daniel, 'Look you don't want to take any notice of all that rubbish on telly. It's a load of bloody nonsense. Half the stuff is done for dramatic effect to put the viewer ratings up. You just have to focus on what this operation could do for you, and go for it.'

Emma broke in before Sara could get any further. 'Daniel, I think the next step is for you to have some time to think about what you'd like to ask, and then you and I can meet up tomorrow and take it from there,' she said.

Sara started to argue and for a few moments everyone was talking at once, until Susan's voice cut through the rest. 'Please. PLEASE! I don't think I can take this anymore.' Everyone fell silent, and she went on quietly, 'Sara this is the way they do things here, and Emma's right. We must let Daniel have some time to decide.'

Reasons to be fearful

'So have you had a chance to think about things – about what you'd like to ask?' Emma said the next day, when she and Daniel were alone together.

'Yeah, I've thought about it quite a bit. To be honest, I'm not sure that I want this transplant.'

'Is there anything particular that's frightening you, Daniel?' Emma asked.

'Needles,' Daniel said immediately. 'I know that sounds pathetic, but if they have to take my portacath out, I'll have to have needles again, and that really freaks me out.'

'Daniel, I do understand that, and it's not pathetic. Many young people in your position get phobic about needles, and we have lots of ways to help you with that. Believe me, we really can make that part much easier for you.'

'There's another thing that may sound daft,' Daniel said hesitantly. 'About the lungs . . .' He tailed off, obviously having trouble continuing, but eventually he went on. 'Could they come from . . . well, from a girl? Because they have a lot of oestrogen, don't they? I was talking to a mate and he said that if I get lungs from a girl I could grow breasts.'

This was a surprisingly common question. Some of Daniel's anxiety went beyond the question of breasts to a more fundamental anxiety about identity. 'One thing I can absolutely promise you, Daniel,' Emma said gently. 'If you were to be transplanted from a female donor you wouldn't grow breasts. You would still be you.'

'What about the donor's family?' Daniel asked. 'If they wanted to meet me, would I have to do that? Because I really don't think I could face all that.'

'No, you wouldn't have to meet them – in fact, it's not something we encourage at all. But if you wanted to send an anonymous letter, that would be fine, and we could help you with that.'

There was a long pause, and Emma asked, 'Were there other things you wanted to ask, Daniel?'

'No, not really,' Daniel replied. 'You see, I have read a lot of that stuff that Sara printed off the Internet, and sometimes I do think beyond the transplant to all the good stuff. You know, being able to get out and do things again. But inside . . . well, I know this sounds a bit crazy – but I think I'm going to die. I have this feeling that I won't make it. That something will go wrong and my body will reject it. If that happens, it's not like a kidney transplant, where you can go back on dialysis. It's the end of the line then.

Then the other thing that Sara doesn't like to talk about is that at best this is only going to buy me a few years. Kids don't normally survive more than a few years after these transplants, do they? It could be a lot of pain and grief for not much time.

'That's true Daniel. But we are getting better at this all the time, and the survival data is improving every year.'

'It's just so hard, you know. You see, my mother, she's been very depressed. She's on pills for it. It makes it really difficult for me to talk to her about all this. If I told her what I told you just now, it'd be like turning a tap on. It's bad enough, even on a good day. I think we're pushing up shares in Kleenex.' He tried to smile at Emma, then looked down quickly and picked at a seam on his trainer, while he fought back his own tears. 'Then there's Sara – well, she's a real hard nut. Everything is so simple for her, and she gets cross with me because she thinks I'm being a coward about this.'

'I know it's hard, Daniel,' Emma said. 'Your mum and Sara both love you so much, and they're just showing it in different ways. What about your dad? I know you still see quite a bit of him. Is he someone you can talk to?'

'Yeah, my dad's alright. He's really bad about hospitals and medical stuff, so he didn't want to come in here with us. But it is easier to talk to another bloke about things. I'm going to stay with him next weekend. Would I be able to wait 'til after that before we make a decision?'

'Daniel, of course,' Emma said. 'You can take as long as you need.'

Daniel was silent for a long time, and Emma wondered whether he had had enough for one day. But she sensed there was something still unsaid, so she sat quietly and waited.

'You said that it's an average of twelve to eighteen months until people get a transplant didn't you?' Daniel said eventually. Emma nodded. 'Well averages are made of shorts and longs,' Daniel continued. 'It could be two years, it could be three years, I might never get that transplant.'

'That's true Daniel. I really wish I could promise you that you'll get to the top of the list – but you know I can't.'

'You see, this may sound a bit weird to you, but if I come to terms with the fact that I'm going to die, I feel as if I can be in control. I'll know what's going to happen and I can be ready for it. But if I go on that list . . . well, all the time I'll be waiting and hoping. Waiting for that phone to ring. Every day just hoping. It's the hoping that really frightens me.'

Eventually he couldn't hold the tears back any longer. 'Did you ever see *The Shawshank Redemption*?' he asked suddenly. Emma was a bit taken aback by the knight's move, but admitted that yes, she had.

'You know what Morgan Freeman said in that movie? He said, "Hope can drive a man insane". And it's true.'

Cut! Rewind

Daniel was fifteen years old. He should have been making decisions about whether he wanted to stay on at school after his GCSEs and what job he might do when he grew up. Instead he was faced with the decision of whether to put his name on the waiting list for a heart–lung transplant – a life-and-death gamble that no fifteen-year-old should have to confront. Was he competent to make such a decision, or was it up to his family and the transplant team to make it for him? What if his decision was different from his parents' – or from that of the doctors and nurses looking after him? Who had the right to decide?

Supporting patients and families through difficult decisions such as this is the ultimate test of every system and every value-set underlying current practice in the NHS. True informed consent is the hallmark of whether we have achieved a shift from paternalism to patient empowerment. It is dependent on the clinical team being able to communicate the risks and benefits effectively, on real sharing of information, on time, on resources and on mutual respect and trust. This can be hard enough when the risk-benefit balance is clear and the patient is an adult, but is inevitably harder still when the risk-benefit balance is unclear, the patient is a child and the decision is a life-and-death one.

In this chapter, I will discuss some of the legal and ethical frameworks underlying these complex issues, and how the frameworks have changed over the past few years. The issue of patient autonomy and choice has risen up the political and social agenda, as the outcome of a changing relationship between the public, the Government and health-care professionals. Clinicians cannot remain immune to the demands and pressures of this changing relationship, and I will discuss the impact of shared decisions on all those 'at the front line' – patients and staff alike – and highlight some of the challenges for all concerned.

THE HEALTH-CARE SYSTEM: COMPETENCE AND INFORMING CONSENT

In Chapter 6, I discussed the systems for evaluating the diagnostic tests, treatments and care plans that we offer to patients, and the way in which we share information about those clinical options. The final, but crucial, aspect of the health-care system is the legal and ethical framework within which patients and staff come together to make decisions about treatment plans: the process of consent.

'Consent' is a patient's agreement for a health professional to provide care. Patients may indicate consent non-verbally (for example, by presenting their arm for their pulse to be taken), orally or in writing. For the consent to be valid, the patient must:

- be competent to take the particular decision;
- have received sufficient information to take it;
- not be acting under duress.

(Department of Health 2001c)

Competence

Competence is an essential prerequisite to consent. A person who is not competent may agree to a treatment, but they cannot give formal consent. How do we know if a patient is competent? There is no single test that determines competence; it is situation-specific and can be complex and difficult to assess, particularly in children.

Competence in adults

Adults are presumed to be competent unless demonstrated otherwise and cannot be treated against their wishes; to do so constitutes battery. The legal test of competence was established by Justice Thorpe in *Re C* (1994). Mr C was a schizophrenic patient in a psychiatric hospital who had the delusion that he was a world-famous doctor. He developed gangrene of the right foot and refused consent to amputation, although the doctors deemed that without this, his chances of survival were small. Despite his delusional state, he was still considered competent to make a decision about his treatment, based on the following provisions (since termed the 'Re C test') (Tan and McMillan 2004: 427):

An adult has capacity to consent (or refuse consent) to medical treatment if he or she can:

- understand and retain information relevant to the decision
- believe that information
- weigh that information in the balance to arrive at a choice.

(Justice Thorpe in *Re C*, 1994)

This legal position stems from the basic right of autonomy and self-determination – the right of the individual to live according to his or her personal choices. John Stuart Mill, in his famous essay 'On Liberty', argues that the only justification for overriding that right is to prevent the individual doing harm to others (Mill 1859: 515). It may well be hard for those charged with the preservation of life to understand and accept that a patient's choice does not have to be in his or her own best interests, or even to be rational by the standards of the majority, as outlined in Lord Donaldson's judgement below:

An adult patient who suffers from no mental incapacity has an absolute right to choose whether to consent to medical treatment, to refuse it, or to choose one rather than another of the treatments being offered [. . .] This right of choice is not limited to decisions which others might regard as sensible. It exists notwithstanding that the reasons for making the choice are rational, irrational, unknown or even non-existent.

(Lord Donaldson in *Re T*, 1992)

Paternalism and autonomy do not make compatible bedfellows. In law, acting in a patient's interests may mean supporting his or her right to self-determination, even in a situation where this could result in death. An adult Jehovah's Witness has the right to refuse blood transfusion, regardless of the consequences, provided that he or she is competent. The right of the individual is paramount, and it is only if the patient's wishes are in doubt that the clinician can err in favour of preserving life. Even if a patient is no longer competent, there is an obligation to try and determine what his or her wishes would have been, whether from an advance statement – also termed a living will (which states how a patient would like to be treated in the event that they lose capacity) – or from a relative.

The only circumstance in which a clinician can act in the 'best interests' of a patient without obtaining consent is if that patient is temporarily or permanently incompetent. For example, a patient may be unconscious, or may be suffering from temporary or permanent mental incapacity. In an emergency, a clinician may intervene to preserve life or take other urgent measures on behalf of the patient and, indeed, has a duty to do so. In a non-urgent situation, the decision about what is in the best interests of the patient may extend beyond purely medical issues to broader social and personal issues. Collaborative decision-making, with the patient's family and, where necessary, with the support of a clinical ethics committee and through application to the courts, is essential.

> It is, I think, important that there should not be a belief that what the doctor says is in the patient's best interest is the patient's best interest. For my part, I would certainly reserve to the Court the ultimate power and duty to review the doctor's discretion in the light of all the facts.
>
> (Sir Thomas Binham in *Frenchay Healthcare NHS Trust* v. *S*, 1994)

Box 7.1 Learning points for clinicians and patients: competence in adults

- No one can give consent on behalf of a competent adult.
- The right to self-determination takes precedence over the sanctity of life.
- Every effort should be made to determine the prior wishes of an incompetent patient.
- 'Best interests' judgements can only be made if the patient's own wishes are in doubt.

continued

- A clinician can and should act in an emergency to preserve life if a patient is temporarily incompetent.
- In decisions about treatment of an incompetent patient, the court should be involved if there is doubt about the course of action that serves the best interests of the patient.

Competence in children

Competence in children is an even more complex issue than competence in adults. In law, children are those under eighteen years old. The law varies, depending on the age of the child.

Consent to treatment

The Family Law Reform Act 1969 (s8) allows children of sixteen or seventeen years to consent to treatment in the same way as an adult (but see below regarding refusal of treatment). For children under the age of sixteen, a child is able to consent to treatment if they are deemed 'Gillick' or 'Fraser' competent.

The Gillick case was precipitated by a Department of Health and Social Security circular that allowed doctors to prescribe contraceptives for a girl under sixteen. Although the recommendation was that girls should be encouraged to inform and consult their parents, they were under no obligation to do so. In response to this circular, Victoria Gillick, a mother of five girls under the age of thirteen, brought an action against her local area health authority, seeking a declaration that the circular was unlawful (*Gillick* v. *West Norfolk and Wisbech Health Authority*, 1985). The case went to the House of Lords, which found in favour of the Health Authority. The key statements and guidance on the case were given by Lords Scarman and Fraser:

> Provided the patient, whether a boy or a girl, is capable of understanding what is proposed, and of expressing his or her own wishes, I see no good reason for holding that he or she lacks the capacity to express them validly and effectively and to authorise the medical man to make the examination or give the treatment which he advises.
>
> (Lord Fraser in *Gillick* v. *West Norfolk and Wisbech Health Authority*, 1985)

The parental right to determine whether or not their minor child below the age of 16 will have medical treatment terminates if and when the child achieves sufficient understanding and intelligence to enable him to understand fully what is proposed.

(Lord Scarman in *Gillick* v. *West Norfolk and Wisbech Health Authority*, 1985)

In effect, this means that although doctors should make every attempt to involve a parent in the decision-making process, a child under sixteen can give consent if he or she understands the nature, purpose and possible consequences of the treatment proposed, the other options and the consequences of not having the treatment. There is no stipulation that the child's decision has to be a wise one, but the Children Act (1989) places an obligation on the clinician to act in the best interests of the child.

Making judgements about whether a child is Gillick-competent can be very difficult. Children vary enormously in their maturity and understanding. There are also differences between boys and girls; for example, one study found that girls and their parents felt confident about their ability to make decisions about surgery two years earlier than boys and their parents (at thirteen compared to fifteen) (Shaw 2001: 150).

Refusal of treatment

There is a major paradox in the application of the law governing consent in children. The courts apply the same criteria to establish understanding in adolescents as they do in adults, but do so in a manner that is entirely at odds with the key features of the adult test outlined previously. The legal position was established through two judgements: one concerning a fifteen-year-old girl refusing antipsychotic medication, and the other a sixteen-year-old girl refusing treatment for anorexia. In both cases, the child's refusal of treatment was overruled. This means that for children under eighteen there are two 'keys' to allow treatment to proceed: consent can be given by the parent or the competent child. Conversely, a child's refusal can be vetoed by their parents if that refusal will lead to death or severe permanent injury.

This position has been upheld in every case that has gone to court, on the basis that the children were not competent. For example,

Re L (1998) concerned a fourteen-year-old girl who had sustained extensive and severe burns and needed blood transfusion. She was a Jehovah's Witness and had signed two advance directives. When the case went to court, it was concluded that she had led a very sheltered life, had limited understanding and experience and seemed to be hoping for a miracle; hence she was not deemed Gillick competent. Re E (1993) concerned another Jehovah's Witness aged fifteen and three-quarters who did not want a life-saving blood transfusion (Enright 2004). The boy was not deemed competent to withhold his consent because, although he was aware that death would follow upon his refusal, he did not understand the horrendous way in which his death would occur. However, since he had never been told, by either the judge or the doctors, exactly what his death would involve, he had effectively been rendered incompetent by having information withheld. Variations on these arguments have been applied in several other cases in which children were deemed incompetent to refuse treatment. In short, the law will resort to any argument possible to avoid allowing an adolescent to refuse life-saving treatment.

Box 7.2 Learning points for clinicians and patients: when can children give consent?

- In law, adulthood begins at age eighteen.
- The Family Law Reform Act (1969) allows children of sixteen or seventeen to give consent in the same way as adults.
- Children under the age of sixteen can give consent if they are Gillick-competent.
- In all cases that have gone to court, no child under the age of eighteen has been successful in refusing life-saving treatment.

> ## Box 7.3 Learning points for clinicians and patients: assessing competence in children
>
> - Ability to understand that there is a choice and that choices have consequences.
> - Willingness and ability to make a choice (including the option of choosing that someone else makes treatment decisions).
> - Understanding of the nature and purpose of the procedure.
> - Understanding of the procedure's risks and side effects.
> - Understanding of the alternatives to the procedure and the risks attached to them, and the consequences of no treatment.
> - Freedom from pressure.
>
> (British Medical Association and Law Society 1995)

What might this mean for Daniel if he decides that he does not want to go ahead with the transplant? There is a possible parallel in the case of Re M (1999), who was a competent fifteen-and-a-half-year-old who sustained acute heart failure and required a heart transplant. She stated that she did not want someone else's heart and refused to give consent. It was considered to be in her best interests to have the transplant and (although she ultimately consented to the operation) it is clear that treatment would have been declared lawful despite a refusal.

In fact, Daniel's case is more complicated than many of those that have gone to court, because in Daniel's situation the risk-benefit balance of the transplant is not as clear-cut. It is much harder to justify compelling a mature minor to have a treatment where there may be limited success or the treatment itself may be painful or distressing (Hagger 2004: 460). Of course, there is no way that the transplant team would suggest that Daniel should have a transplant unless they felt that there was a good chance of increasing the length and quality of his life, but there is the inescapable and not insignificant risk that he could die during or shortly after the operation. In theory, a child's refusal for treatment can be overridden by just one parent. So if either Susan or Matthew gave consent for the transplant – even if the other refused – this would still be valid. In practice, the transplant team would do all in their power to help the family arrive at a consensus view. It is very doubtful that they would consider it to be in Daniel's best interests to force a transplant on him if, say, both he and Susan refused, and Matthew consented. The most important task for the team, therefore, is to ensure that Daniel and his family can make a properly informed decision that they can all feel confident is the right one.

Informing consent

We have established that valid consent requires capacity and freedom from duress. The third and most critical part of the consent requirement is information. Until relatively recently, the process of obtaining consent consisted all too frequently of the most junior member of the medical team thrusting a piece of paper into the hands of the patient, running through the details of the procedure in a perfunctory and incomplete manner and securing a signature at the bottom of the page. Much has changed since then, and understanding the importance of properly informed consent has transformed the relationship between patients and clinicians.

Consent is not about the signature on the piece of paper. It is a process of informing and agreeing that takes place between a patient and a clinician – most commonly, a doctor. The NHS Plan highlighted the need for a radical change to the way in which patients are asked to give their consent to treatment, and this was a key theme of the Bristol Royal Infirmary Inquiry (2001) (see later in this chapter). This issue is now of such central importance that guidance can be found from a number of sources including the BMA, the GMC and the Department of Health web sites. The quotes below indicate the fundamental change in our beliefs about patients' rights to information:

> Perform [your duties] calmly and adroitly, concealing most things from the patient while you are attending to him. Give necessary orders with cheerfulness and sincerity, turning his attention away from what is being done to him; sometimes reprove sharply and emphatically, and sometimes comfort with solicitude and attention, revealing nothing of the patient's future or present condition.
>
> (Hippocrates, circa 400 BC, from
> Teuten and Taylor 2001: 894)

> A surgeon owes a legal duty to a patient to warn him or her in general terms of possible serious risks involved in the procedure [. . .] In modern law medical paternalism no longer rules and a patient has a prima facie right to be informed by a surgeon of a small, but well established, risk of serious injury as a result of surgery.
>
> (Lord Steyn in *Chester* v. *Afshar*, 2004)

Although Hippocrates was writing 2,500 years ago, this change in attitude is a relatively recent phenomenon. Only fifty years ago, in 1954, a BBC broadcaster presented with a nodule on her thyroid gland. When surgical removal was recommended, she asked if the operation posed any threat to her voice, and was reassured. Surgery proceeded and a nerve was damaged during the operation. As a result she could no longer speak properly, and the case went to court. Lord Justice Denning found in favour of the doctor, on the basis that lying to the patient about the true risk of surgery was justified by the need to protect her from worry (Teuten and Taylor 2001: 894).

What do patients need and want to know in order to make an informed choice? Clearly, a doctor discussing a possible surgical procedure with a patient is not going to give a history of all the different surgical techniques that have been used, the results of all the papers on the subject and a detailed account of the minutiae of the operation. Inevitably, the doctor will put a filter on the information that the patient receives. That filter should include all the information that might be relevant to the patient's decision about whether or not to proceed – and different patients will need different filters. One of the most difficult skills in modern medicine is listening carefully to what patients want to know and providing enough information to ensure that their decisions are based on a full understanding of the facts. How to achieve this without making paternalistic judgements about the sharing of information?

The GMC and BMA have produced guidance on the sort of information that doctors should provide. The following is a summary of some of the key points:

Box 7.4 Learning points for clinicians: information that should be provided to patients planning to undergo a treatment or procedure

- The purpose of the treatment, and likely benefits.
- The strength of the evidence supporting the proposed treatment, and its applicability to the patient's condition.
- Other options for treatment, including the option not to treat.
- The likely benefits and probabilities of success for each option.
- Known possible risks and side effects.
- Lifestyle changes that may be caused or necessitated by the treatment.
- How the patient's condition and any side effects will be monitored.
- The possibility of additional problems coming to light during the procedure or treatment, and possible action in this event.
- The name of the doctor who will have overall responsibility.
- A reminder that the patient can change his or her mind at any time.

Consent covers a wide variety of procedures in medicine, including screening, use of diagnostic tests and treatment. However, the majority of problems arise because a patient feels that risks were not disclosed or adequately explained. One of the landmark cases was *Sidaway* v. *Board of Governors of the Bethlem Royal Hospital* in 1985. In this case, the House of Lords rejected the patient's claim that a surgeon was negligent in not disclosing the risk of spinal-cord damage, which she subsequently sustained. Their decision was based on the premise that a reasonable body of neurosurgeons in that position would not have disclosed the risk (in other words, their judgement was based on the Bolam test, see Chapter 5).

Since *Sidaway*, the courts have adopted a more patient-centred approach to consent, through which some key principles have emerged: first, that a doctor is under an obligation to tell the truth if asked a direct question by a patient (*Rogers* v. *Whittaker*, 1992) and, second, to warn of a 'significant risk that would affect the decision of a reasonable patient' (*Pearce* v. *United Bristol Healthcare NHS Trust*, 1999). The problem is that there are no hard and fast rules as to what constitutes a significant risk that would affect the decision of a reasonable patient. A figure of 1–2 per cent is often quoted, but is not set in any definitive guidance.

More recently, the situation has become even more complicated as a result of a subtle but important change through the case of *Chester* v. *Afshar* (2004). The quote from Lord Steyn, cited above, was drawn from this case, in which Mr Afshar, the surgeon, failed to warn Miss Chester of a 1–2 per cent risk of paralysis following surgery for back pain. In this instance, the Law Lords found in favour of the patient, even though Miss Chester did not make any claim that had she been warned of the risk, she would have changed her decision about having the surgery. It is rather ironic that this significant change has come through such a similar set of clinical circumstances to that of *Sidaway*.

What does all this mean in practice? At present, it is too early to fully assess the impact of *Chester* v. *Afshar*, so doctors will need to act on well-established principles. A good starting point is the GMC's advice to start the consent process with an exploration of the patient's objectives (Bridson et al. 2003: 1159). Often, those objectives will be framed in terms of social rather than medical outcomes, such as surviving until a family wedding, being able to take a child to school or being able to take part in a sporting activity. The Australian Law Reform Commission (1989) is more explicit about how to approach patient-centred consent and recommends that clinicians take account of factors such as the patient's temperament, understanding, desire for information, the nature of the treatment, the magnitude of possible harm and the likelihood of risk. Ultimately, the process of consent is dependent on a combination of trust, judgement, shared understanding, time and communication. In the absence of prescriptive rules, clinicians have to continue to do their best to get this right, whilst acknowledging that the consent process itself is as fallible as the medical procedures for which consent is sought.

THE SOCIETAL CONTEXT: 'ALL CHANGED, CHANGED UTTERLY'

So wrote Richard Smith, Editor of the *BMJ*, quoting W. B. Yeats in an editorial published in the week after judgement was passed on the Bristol case (Smith 1998: 1917). He described the case as a once-in-a-lifetime drama and predicted that it that would be more important to the future of health care than White Papers and NHS reorganisations.

> At the heart of the tragedy . . . is 'the trust that patients place in their doctors'. That trust will never be the same again, but that will be a good thing if we move to an active rather than a passive trust, where doctors share uncertainty.
>
> (Smith 1998: 1917)

I referred briefly to the Bristol case in Chapter 1, but it is important to expand on the key facts. The four key figures in the drama were James Wisheart, who was cardio-thoracic surgeon, Director of Cardiac Services and subsequently Medical Director at Bristol Royal Infirmary; Janardan Dhasmana, a cardiothoracic surgeon in the unit led by Wisheart; John Roylance, Chief Executive of the trust and a radiologist by background; and a young anaesthetist called Stephen Bolsin. In 1988 when Stephen Bolsin joined the team, there were already worrying figures emerging that suggested that the mortality of babies having cardiac surgery at Bristol was twice the national average. In 1990 Bolsin wrote to Roylance, expressing his concerns, but was referred back to Wisheart – one of the surgeons carrying out the operations. In 1994, a new professor of cardiac surgery was appointed and, after reviewing the data, he recommended that complex cardiac surgery on young babies should be stopped. In 1995, in the face of this agreed cessation of surgery, a decision was made to operate on Joshua Loveday, following a special meeting chaired by James Wisheart. Janardan Dhasmana operated, and Joshua died. It was this death that finally brought the tragedy to public attention.

There were many failings identified through the subsequent inquiry – failings that were symptomatic of the NHS at that time, including lack of dedicated paediatric intensive-care beds, a shortage of trained nurses, poor teamwork and an inadequate understanding of the essentials of care for sick children. However, Wisheart, Roylance and Dhasmana were all found to be personally culpable to a greater or lesser degree – both by the inquiry and by the GMC. Their guilt lay not in failings of technical or clinical performance, but in lack of insight, in a 'club culture', in failures of communication and, ultimately, therefore, in betrayal of trust.

Trust and communication have been recurring themes throughout this book. In Chapter 3 I discussed the trust that patients place in individual clinicians and in their health-care teams. Trust is eroded by medical error and uncertainty, yet it is an essential commodity in joint decision-making. I developed these themes through Chapters 5 and 6, and in this chapter described how consent – particularly in high-stake situations – is the ultimate test of trust and good communication.

Richard Smith feared that the trust that underpins the relationship between individual patients and their doctors would be a casualty of Bristol, alongside a broader loss of trust in the medical profession. He has been proved both right and wrong in his predictions: right in predicting that the impact of Bristol would be more far-reaching and profound than that of government White Papers; wrong in predicting damage to individual doctor–patient relationships. The MORI data cited in Chapter 2 confirm that despite the damaging medical scandals, patients do still trust their doctors, but they expect very different doctors from the paternalistic figures that have held sway since the birth of the NHS.

Sir Donald Irvine, in *The Doctor's Tale* (Irvine 2003), described the more unhelpful 'tribal' characteristics of the medical profession that have evolved over the past few decades. These characteristics and attitudes were the soil in which the Bristol tragedy would take root. They include:

A culture of elitism, founded on high performance as a diagnostician/technician/scientist, which [. . .] came to dominate the medical schools, especially in the early years of the NHS. This culture, to which all students were exposed, had obvious strengths but was dismissive of failure. Sir Lancelot Spratt, the grand surgeon in the book and film *Doctor in the House* was the caricature based on reality.

A profession whose outward reputation is dependent on [. . .] being right, yet has to handle the serious stresses and strains on individuals who may feel torn between preserving their reputation and revealing their own feelings of fallibility or uncertainty.

A relative lack of attention to personal attitudes and conduct, particularly in matters of consent and communication with patients and their relatives, which simply fuels the perception of a doctor as paternalistic, detached or arrogant.

(Irvine 2003: 25)

Although much of the post-Bristol debate has been about the ability of the medical profession to self-regulate, achievement of a regulatory framework will ultimately be a matter of process. In the light of Dame Janet Smith's report (see Chapter 2), the development of that process may have some way to go, but procedures will be established independently of any need for active involvement of the majority of the medical profession or the public – and doctors will comply with them. However, the more transformational impact of the Bristol affair is its impact on the culture of medical paternalism.

Paternalism, partnership and patient choice

The shift from paternalism to partnership is dependent on a recognition that both the clinician and the patient are experts in their own right – and that both have responsibilities in the process of agreeing treatment plans (Coulter 1999: 719). In a doctor–patient partnership, the doctor is knowledgeable about diagnosis, treatment options, risk and prognosis, and the patient is knowledgeable about his or her experience of illness, social circumstances, attitudes to risk and preferences. Information-sharing has to be a two-way process, in order to be most effective, and both parties have to be prepared to take the other's concerns seriously.

Towle and Godolphin (1999: 766) have tried to explore the skills that both patients and doctors need in order to arrive at shared decisions. The challenge for doctors is that they make assumptions and inaccurate guesses about patients' concerns, and this can lead to misunderstandings and a failure to provide the information that the patient wants and needs. An alarming statistic is that most doctors interrupt patients less than half a minute into the consultation (Marvel et al. 1999: 283) – so small wonder that they may not always develop an adequate grasp of their agenda. Yet it has been shown that the consultation does not take any longer if the patient is allowed to fully express his or her concerns. In fact, conversely, it can be concluded more rapidly and with a more satisfactory outcome.

In Chapter 2 I discussed how easy it is for clinicians to fall into the trap of giving premature or inappropriate reassurance, rather than eliciting the patient's real concerns. It was very clear by Chapter 6 that Susan had serious worries about Daniel's deteriorating lung function, but she was unable to express them in her consultation with Sebastian Hill and Mo Khan. For practical purposes, Sebastian and Mo had decided on the 'correct' course of action before Susan and Daniel walked through the door and were very focused on starting him on a trial of azithromicin. They minimised any concerns about side effects or the possibility that it wouldn't work, and what they achieved was 'informed compliance' rather than informed consent, with little real opportunity for negotiation.

Many medical consultations proceed in this way and, although enabling the patient to take a more active role will not always lead to a different outcome in terms of treatment decisions, it will lead to a greater sense of ownership. Importantly, if the clinician is able to respond to cues expressed in a variety of verbal and non-verbal ways, there will be occasions when the patient makes quite different choices. For example, in this chapter we saw how astute Emma was in responding to Daniel's cues – even when those cues were silence or diffidence. Jean Simons (Assistant Director of Family Policy at GOSH) leads on teaching staff across the hospital how to improve their interactive communication and how to support shared decision-making. Figure 7.1, produced by Jean Simons, is part of a broader communication-skills training and assessment package that she is developing. It highlights the difference between informed compliance and informed consent and summarises some of the issues that have been discussed above and throughout earlier parts of this book.

On the flip side, patients need an array of skills as well. Those who are most active in managing their health and illness also have active strategies for managing their doctors (Towle and Godolphin

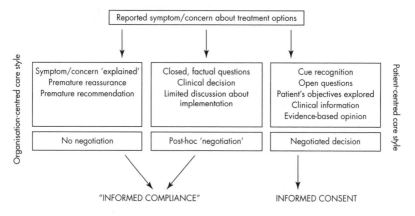

Figure 7.1 Shared decision-making.

Reproduced with kind permission from Jean Simons.

1999: 766). Being an 'expert' autonomous patient is no mean feat (Jadad et al. 2003: 1293) – especially when you are ill. The 'ideal' autonomous patient of the future will bring a list of questions to the consultation, will know how involved he or she wants to be in health-care decisions, will have a file of up-to-date information from all key professionals involved in his or her care, will have Internet access and the ability to filter large volumes of information in order to present the health-care professional with a distillation of concerns and queries. In the past, health professionals had to cope with information overload, while patients had to cope with information deficit (Eysenbach and Jadad 2001: E19). Now patients have opportunities to access information in abundance, through mass media, self-support groups and, particularly, the Internet. The problem is that the Internet gives unlimited access to poorly organised information, with no quality control, and no means of assessing the source and calibre (see Chapters 2 and 6).

Despite the hurdles, many patients can and do manage this medley of tasks and skills. Some cannot – or choose not to do so. In part, this may be an age-related phenomenon, with younger patients being more ready to challenge medical paternalism and more able to access information. However, at the point of vulnerability, not all patients want to take the full burden of responsibility for their illness. There is a spectrum of how much control and information individual patients wish to have, and doctors have to be sensitive to these preferences as much as to clear treatment preferences. The medical profession did not nurture and develop paternalism single-handedly; it is a two-way street. If the public wants to see an end to medical paternalism, a two-way contract of participation and responsibility has to be established.

AT THE FRONT LINE: JUNIOR PARTNERS

From adolescence to autonomy

The challenges to shared decision-making and partnership are considerable when the patient is an adult. Daniel was at the threshold of adulthood. He was at that most difficult time, when adolescents are normally developing a personal identity to enhance their independence. Acting out, living dangerously and taking risks are a normal part of that process, but these were luxuries that Daniel could ill afford in his compromised state of health. He had to contend with a chronic illness that made him different from his peers, a mother who was depressed and understandably anxious about letting go, a sister who was trying to speak for him and an absent father – and, on top of all that and the day-to-day burdens of his treatment, a life-and-death decision as well.

Identity, risk and non-adherence to treatment

Adolescence is a time when it is normal to challenge authority. Adolescents with chronic illnesses are adolescents first and ill second. Their need to challenge is just as great as that of their peers. Although chronically sick teenagers are less likely to indulge in risky behaviour, that is not to say that they won't take risks. For example, in a study by Tyrrell (2001: 139), 21 per cent of teenagers with cystic fibrosis smoked, compared to 56 per cent of controls.

One way in which adolescents with a chronic illness can assert their authority and independence is by rebelling against their treatment. Non-adherence to treatment (or 'non-compliance') is extremely common. Given that it is almost impossible to get an adolescent to comply with day-to-day requests such as keeping their room tidy or coming home on time, why on earth would it be possible to get them to comply with inconvenient, difficult or distressing treatment regimes? 'Defiance' rather than 'compliance' is likely to be the norm.

When adolescents fail to comply with treatment, it is rarely because they've made an active decision that it's not the right therapy for them or because they are concerned about side effects. More often the drivers are much more straightforward and practical: it's too time-consuming, too stigmatising, too disruptive, and they've had enough. Children with chronic disorders face heavy burdens: long-term, complex treatments that constantly remind them that they are ill, different from their peers, may have progressive complications and may possibly die young.

The following strategies may help improve adherence to treatment:

Box 7.5 Learning points for clinicians and parents: improving adherence to treatment in adolescents

- Children who have medical conditions often feel disempowered; letting them make decisions from an early age which do not ultimately carry much weight gives them, and you, a chance to explore letting go safely.
- Gradually increase involvement in treatment over time. Adolescents who are independent in their treatment are also independent in other aspects of their lives.
- Be as flexible about treatment plans as possible, and try to think 'out of the box'. Joining a gym may be a substitute for some physiotherapy sessions. Where possible, allow the adolescent some freedom to plan drug regimes, admissions and other aspects of treatment.
- If youngsters are really at the end of their tether, build in 'treatment holidays' where possible. It is better to do this as an agreed plan than for the adolescent to do it in a more risky way.
- Make it possible for them to admit they are not fully complying with treatment by acknowledging how difficult compliance is. 'How many times did you manage to do your treatment this week?', is better than 'Have you done all your treatments this week?'
- Be aware of other stressors, apart from the illness itself, which may contribute to depression or non-compliance.
- Support from other youngsters, or sometimes older people with the same condition, can be helpful.

(Adapted from Michaud et al. 2004: 943, Tyrrell 2001: 139)

Consultations and meetings

As children get older, they will gradually move on to the stage where they take full responsibility for their care. In time, that will include attending outpatient appointments by themselves. At an earlier stage, they may wish to be copied in to letters. Timing of this will vary considerably, depending on their maturity and wishes and the views of their family.

Depending on their illness, they may need to attend larger meetings – as Daniel had to in thinking about his transplant decision. When planning larger meetings involving older children and adolescents, it is very important to consider their needs. Children with disabilities may have particular needs (for example, physical needs, visual or hearing impairments, and so on). Participation is not just about having the child in the room – it is a more active process.

Box 7.6 Learning points for clinicians and parents: meetings involving older children and adolescents

- Prepare in advance. Tell the child or adolescent who will be there, what the purpose of the meeting will be and be honest about how much influence he or she will have on the decision (Sinclair and Franklin 2000).
- Take account of the young person's agenda and make sure enough time is given to his or her concerns.
- Rethink the style of the meeting. Large meetings with complex discussions can be intimidating. Think carefully about who and what is needed (Sinclair and Franklin 2000).
- Treat the young person with respect and make sure their contribution is listened to and given weight and credibility.
- Be very clear about what will happen next.

Difficult decisions

There are no easy answers as to how best to support children and families through difficult decisions. Experience and time are both important commodities. The following pointers may be helpful:

Box 7.7 Learning points for clinicians: supporting young people and families through difficult decisions

- It is very important to give children and families all the time they need to talk and ask questions, in person or on the phone, when they are considering difficult decisions.
- Children may disagree with their parents or other family members about treatment options. Every effort should be made to bring them to consensus. Occasionally, this will not be possible. Both group and individual meetings may be needed.
- Be careful not to listen most attentively to the loudest voices. The quiet child may have a lot to talk about.
- If a child's reaction to a suggested treatment plan is initially hostile, this may reflect as yet unexpressed anxieties. Children of all ages may need frequent chances to talk to the professionals on a one-to-one basis.
- Parents may, understandably, want to protect their child from unpleasant truths, such as that they are dying. This may not be in the child's best interests and it is important to understand why parents feel this way.
- Parents may be reluctant to talk to their children because they themselves are too emotional. Again, offering them lots of time and support, in person and on the phone, is essential.
- Some children feel the same way and find it difficult to talk to their parents. Professional time and support can help.
- Turning down treatment is a valid choice. Professionals may disagree but must respect this, if it is the considered decision of the child and family, and must continue to provide support, except in exceptional circumstances, as described in the previous legal precedents.

Supporting parents in 'letting go'

Much is written about the difficult transitional issues for adolescents with chronic illnesses. Far less is written about their parents. The process of transition can be just as hard for them as for their children

– particularly when they have devoted many years to their care, sometimes at enormous personal cost. It can be particularly difficult to stay on the sidelines and tolerate non-compliant behaviour after working hard over such an extended period to proactively manage the illness and minimise risk. The following suggestions were written by Bea Teuten, parent and PALS advocate at GOSH:

Box 7.8 Learning points for parents: 'letting go'

- Letting go is a gradual process: recognise the milestones.
- Try to see your child as the individual he or she has become.
- Don't see their decisions, if they differ from your choices, as a rejection of you.
- Try to recognise that it is your hard work and investment that have given them the tools to tackle the huge issues they face.
- All teenagers want to break away.
- Maintain a dialogue; at least that way you will be able to understand how they have reached their choices.
- If you feel they are making the wrong decisions, tell them gently why you disagree and give them time to think about what you have said.
- If necessary, suggest they speak to someone who is less emotionally involved than you are – possibly a family friend or a trusted professional.
- Children often try to protect those they love – try to remember they may be trying to protect you as much as you are trying to protect them.
- Try to remember that every parent has to let go at some stage – and that children who have had to face huge treatment decisions often have an understanding way beyond their years.

Supporting staff

Finally, having spoken about adolescents and their families, it is important not to lose sight of the other people in the partnership: the health-care team. It is unrealistic to talk about partnership and yet assume that the clinical team is immune to any personal engagement and involvement in the outcome of their patients' care. In Daniel's case, the St Michael's and community teams would inevitably be anxious to hear the outcome of his decision about a transplant. Whatever his choice, they would be committed to looking after him through a difficult and stressful time. And, if he decided to go ahead, they would be worried about whether he would survive long enough to get his transplant.

Clinicians live with the 'downstream' impact of decisions made by people whose values and prejudices may differ from their own. They may disagree – or think the patient will later regret their choice – but they still have to give that decision their full support.

How would they cope if Daniel were to decide not to go on the waiting list and then change his mind when it was too late? What if he decided to go on the waiting list and – as he feared – was deteriorating and increasingly unlikely to get a transplant. In that scenario, when would the time be right to discuss what to do if he had a respiratory arrest and needed to be put on a ventilator, knowing that there would be no chance of him coming off again?

Stress among health-care professionals is high, as discussed in Chapter 4. Interestingly, however, counter to what one might predict, palliative-care consultants, who spend their time looking after terminally ill patients, report lower rates of work-related stress and burnout, compared to their colleagues in other specialities (Ramirez et al. 1998: 208). In general, death and dying do not emerge as the main sources of stress in their jobs. Instead they complain of all the same things as other health-care professionals: resource pressures, work–life balance and administrative and management problems. Nonetheless, the death of a young patient, particularly one with whom the professional has formed a close relationship, is more difficult to manage.

There are sources of support for staff, as outlined in Chapter 4. However, these are more generic and are available on a needs-led basis for individual staff members who are experiencing difficulty. It is rare to find support services that work more proactively with clinical teams in known high-stress areas, such as intensive-care units, which have a notoriously high burnout rate (Chen and McMurray 2001: 152).

In the absence of more formal mechanisms, staff utilise other team members as an important source of support. This is another reflection on the importance of good team working. In a health service that cannot afford to lose staff to stress and burnout, more active counselling services may be a sound investment.

At the end of the day

'Come in,' Mo called, in response to the knock on his office door. He had only left the ward ten minutes ago and was intent on getting his clinic letters done, so he hoped this wasn't going to be one of the junior doctors come to tell him about a sick child in A&E. When he saw that it was Penny, he was both pleased and relieved and decided that the clinic letters could wait. He jumped up to move a pile of notes and X-rays off the only other chair in his cupboard-sized room.

'Penny – what a nice surprise,' he said. 'We don't see enough of you these days, now that you're so important. What is it again – Community Children's Services Manager? Do you still have time for a coffee with a humble paediatrician?'

'Love one,' Penny replied, as she sat down. 'And don't give me the humble paediatrician line. I gather you've been talked into taking over as Clinical Director of Women's and Children's Services – so I bet you're just as tied up in management hassles as me.'

'OK, fifteen all,' Mo said and went to make the coffee. When he came back he said, 'You know Patrick Connell died at the weekend?'

'Yes, I dropped into Rainbow on the way up here, and they told me. They were quite upset about it.' Patrick's family were Travellers, and he had had a rare genetic disorder, which had left him with a complex heart problem, seizures, stunted growth and deformed limbs. He had spent much of his life in and out of St Michael's and had died one week short of his third birthday.

'It's always difficult,' Mo said. 'Patrick was a real favourite on the ward, and quite a lot of them want to go to the funeral. Maggie's trying to keep some kind of balance on it – partly to stop them overwhelming the family, and partly because she has to keep the ward staffed.' Penny could sympathise with Maggie, the ward sister. It was a juggling act she had had to manage when she was a ward sister herself. It was always hard to strike the balance between letting the staff have some outlet for their own feelings, showing support for the family and also respecting their right to grieve with some privacy.

'I'm sure my team will be sad as well,' Penny said. 'It's such a shame. He was doing so well after his second operation that I don't think anyone was really prepared for this.'

'I suppose the only thing to say is that his parents had nearly three years that they wouldn't have had a few years back. His cardiac lesion wouldn't even have been operable ten years ago.'

'I know,' Penny said. 'I had a baby with a very similar heart problem. She died at a week old.'

'Oh Penny, I'm so sorry. I had no idea,' Mo said.

'No, don't worry. There's no reason why you should. I don't mention it to many people. My first husband reckoned that I became a nurse to make up for it. I didn't, of course – but there are times when it gives me a perspective I wouldn't otherwise have.'

'I'm sure,' Mo said. 'And I guess times when it makes it harder as well.'

'Yes, maybe,' Penny said, then, after a brief pause, 'On another note, have you heard anything from the Albion about Daniel Johnson? He was up there last week for his transplant assessment, and I haven't caught up with them since.'

'No, I haven't heard yet,' Mo replied. 'So are you still looking after him?'

'Yes, I've kept on a small patient caseload,' Penny said. 'I was just wondering . . . if he decides to go on the transplant waiting list, how would you rate his chances of getting one?'

'Come on, Penny – you know that's an impossible question.'

'Of course it is. But what I'm really asking is how long do you think he'll survive without one?'

'I don't know . . . it's so difficult. I suppose six months . . . certainly not a year.'

'I thought much the same,' Penny said. 'The truth is that I have a horrible feeling that even if he goes through this agonising decision about whether to have a transplant or not, chances are that he won't get one in time.'

'What do you think he will decide, then?' Mo asked.

'I don't know,' Penny said. 'I really just don't know.'

UNRESOLVED QUESTIONS: ORGAN DONATION

UK Transplant is a special health authority within the NHS, with a UK-wide remit for ensuring that donated organs are matched and allocated in a fair and unbiased way. In December 2004, more than 6,000 people on the UK Transplant database were waiting for an organ transplant (UK Transplant 2004a). About 2,800 organs are transplanted each year, but sadly nearly 400 people die each year while waiting for a kidney, lung, heart or liver transplant – and many more die before they even get on to the waiting list. Transplant saves not just lives, but also money. For example, figures from UK Transplant show that a successful kidney transplant will save the NHS approximately 200,000 pounds over ten years, compared to keeping a patient on dialysis over that period. This money can be used to save further lives as it is put back into the Health Service.

Shortage of organs for transplantation is an international problem, and one that has been fiercely and emotively debated across the globe – by the public, by clinicians and by ethicists. Could the supply of organs be increased and what are the ethical and practical issues?

Currently people can become an organ donor in the UK in one of two ways. First, they can be live kidney donors for immediate relatives. Second, they can express their willingness to allow their organs to be used after their death by signing onto the NHS Organ Donor Register or by carrying a donor card. At present, about 20 per cent of the population are registered in this way. However, even when someone has signalled a wish to be an organ donor through the NHS Organ Donor Register, permission to proceed still has to be sought from the next of kin. UK Transplant has been keeping a record of the number of patients who could potentially be organ donors, compared to the number of transplants that actually take place. Between 1 April 2003 and 31 March 2004, there were 1,379 potential donors. A potential donor is someone who is 'brain dead' (medically called 'brain-stem dead'), on intensive care, and who does not have any medical reason not to be able to donate their organs. One hundred and ninety-eight (14 per cent) of the families were not asked about transplant. Of the 1,181 families who were asked, 690 (58 per cent) said 'yes'. One-third of the families who said 'no' were unsure what their relative would have wanted, or were divided about the decision. Religious reasons were given as an objection in only a minority of cases (UK Transplant 2004b).

Two immediate questions spring from this data. First, what are the moral and ethical considerations of introducing a system in which people have to 'opt out' rather than 'opt in' as potential donors? The BMA has taken a strong position in supporting 'presumed consent' for those over the age of sixteen. This view is based on studies that demonstrate that the vast majority of people would be willing to donate their organs, but have neither registered their preference nor discussed it with relatives. If organ donation were the default position, people would have a stronger imperative to discuss their decisions with their families, and it would be much easier to maintain the smaller database of those who wished to opt out for religious or personal reasons. In some parts of Europe, where presumed consent is already in operation, there is preliminary evidence that this has improved transplant rates (Abadie and Gay 2004).

Whatever the likely outcome of public debate about this issue, an even more difficult question follows. Regardless of whether there is a system of presumed consent for transplant, or of 'opting in', as at present, should that consent be 'full' and 'binding'? 'Full' means that once consent has been given (whether presumed or actively), that consent is sufficient and no one else needs to be asked for permission. 'Binding' means that the consent cannot be overridden. Full and binding consent would have two consequences. First, it would address the reluctance of clinicians to discuss organ donation with distressed relatives – a reluctance that is understandable, but that also deprives other patients of the chance of life. Second, it would take away the right of the next of kin to determine the fate of their loved-one's body. If one accepts the principle that every autonomous individual has the right to decide what should happen to his or her body after death, then many would argue that this right should not be overruled by relatives who are uncomfortable with the decision (Kluge 1999: 387). Conversely, there is considerable concern about the prospect of increasing the trauma for bereaved relatives at what is already a deeply distressing time.

As if these questions were not difficult enough, perhaps the greatest controversy relates to the question of buying and selling organs. The topic is a complex and fraught one – so much so that it can be difficult to generate reasoned debate. There is a natural abhorrence to the concept of a market in human organs, and this has been fuelled by the social injustice implicit in rich and privileged individuals being able to obtain organs by 'exploitation' of the poor. Accounts of coercion and profiteering in the developing world and of donor organs being removed in suboptimal medical conditions, have given these anxieties a tangible focus. John Harris is a strong proponent of the need to develop an ethically defensible market in human organs, with built-in safeguards against exploitation (Harris and Erin 2002: 114). His arguments have centred primarily on the creation of a market in organs from the living, although there has also been debate about the possibility of using financial incentives to encourage contracts for organ donation after death. The principles of an ethical market are that there would be a single purchaser (for example, in the UK, this would be the

NHS), and strict financial and quality controls. Arguably only citizens resident in the state or union could sell into the market, in order to remove the possibility of exploitation of low-income countries (Erin and Harris 2003: 137).

Many are opposed to these proposals and, to some degree, the objections spring from a sense of 'moral wrongness' rather than reasoned arguments or clear evidence. Concerns about those 'forced' by poverty to enter such a market do not address the fact that they could be even more disadvantaged if this option was unavailable, and suggestions that a legalised market would reduce the flow of organs from altruistic donation are hypothetical. Outlawing the sale of organs may well make it difficult or impossible for the 'greedy rich' to buy health through this route, but it would be naïve to think that health inequalities can be eliminated by closing this one channel. Short of setting an embargo on private health care and dismantling the entire machinery of privilege (an approach that has been manifestly unsuccessful across the communist states), health inequalities are inherent to our society. The best that can be safeguarded is an equitable minimum standard of care.

The basis on which live donation is sanctioned at all in this country is that the risks are relatively small (a risk of dying during the procedure of 0.03 per cent (Erin and Harris 2003), and a subsequent risk of living with one kidney that is no greater than the risk of driving back and forth to work sixteen miles a day) (Blumstein 1999: 390). Once the principle of live donation is accepted then, regardless of the size of the risk, is it paternalistic and judgemental to impose a value-set that allows donation to a close relative, but does not allow sale for financial benefit? Paul Randall, the father who attempted to sell his kidney to buy therapy for his daughter with cerebral palsy (see Chapter 3, p. 68), would argue that he was trying to use his kidney to improve the quality of his child's life. This aspiration is no different from that of a parent who donates a kidney directly to a son or daughter. There are strong arguments for the right of the individual to choose the risks that they wish to take – be it to go skiing for pleasure, to undertake a job that carries high risk as a trade-off for increased income or to sell an organ. The debate will continue.

**Box 7.9 Learning points for everyone:
        organ donation**

- UK Transplant's web site <http://www.uktransplant.org.
  uk> carries up-to-date information on all aspects of organ
  donation.
- If you want to become an organ donor, you can register on-
  line at UK Transplant, or call the donor line on 0845 60 60
  400.
- For all the reasons outlined above, it is very important to
  discuss your wishes with respect to organ donation with
  your family or next of kin.

8   Endings

When I was a child

'I was just doing my homework in the garden,' Daniel said. 'Come through.'

Penny followed him outside, noticed the Walkman and the unopened maths books, and concluded that not much homework was being done. That was OK.

'Is your mum around?' she asked.

'No, she's nipped out to Tesco. But I'm glad we've got some time to talk,' Daniel said. 'I wanted to tell you. I've decided. Well the truth is, I decided a couple of weeks ago, but I didn't know how to tell people.'

'You're not going to have it,' Penny said. It was a statement, not a question.

'No, I just can't. I'm really sorry Penny.'

'Daniel, please. You don't have to apologise to me, for heaven's sake. It's what's right for you that matters. That's the only thing that's important,' Penny said. Then, unsure whether she was Daniel's first sounding board for this, she said 'Have you told your family yet?'

'Yes, I told them a couple of days ago. I think they were expecting it – like you were. You know at first, after we left the Albion, I tried really hard to be positive. But it's nearly six weeks since the assessment now, and I think they knew that the longer I went on without deciding, the less chance there was that I'd say yes.'

'Are they alright?' Penny asked.

'If you mean, will they go along with what I want, then yes. But they're no way alright – 'specially Mum. I can hardly bear to look at her, because I know she's in tears half the time. She tries not to do it in front of me, but she looks a complete wreck.' After a pause, he went on, 'Anyway, I wanted to tell you why.'

'Daniel, you don't have to justify your decision to me. It's your decision.'

'No, what I mean is I need to tell you. I need to be able to tell someone outside my family – someone who won't burst into tears when I talk about it, and who'll understand. You see, I'm just so tired.'

He was sitting on the edge of the sun lounger, head bowed, but then he looked up at her, and she realised with a jolt that the child she had known was gone. A familiar verse leapt into her head. 'When I was a child, I spoke like a child, I thought like a child, I reasoned like a child. When I became a man, I gave up childish ways.' She pulled her chair closer, and said, 'Go on, Daniel.'

'I really am so tired,' he said again. 'This is just no life. The last year or two, it's been endless. In and out of hospital. The needles, the drugs, the physio, the ward rounds, the tests. Waking up in the morning hardly able to breathe until I've done my physio. I don't want any more of that. I just want it to stop.

'I know I'm just a kid – just fifteen – but I have thought through the implications of this. The thing is, it gets harder and harder seeing all my mates making plans for what they're going to do next year, getting girl-friends, taking off for weekends. It's never going to be like that for me.'

He didn't need her to speak, but he looked at her to read her reaction, and went on, 'It is alright, Penny. I really can come to terms with it now. I can let go because it's so bloody awful. But say I went for it and got the transplant. At best, that would just give me a window of time . . . and then I'd have to face going downhill again. That would be like letting an animal out of a cage, giving it a bit of freedom, then locking it up again. And of course, that's best-case scenario. Chances are I wouldn't even get one anyway.

'The hardest bit is not about me. It's everyone else. I feel like I'm letting everyone down – Mum, Sara, Dad, you, Dr Khan, Dr Stebbing . . . Penny, do you think people will be disappointed in me?'

'No, Daniel. I don't. I think people will be proud of you for making a brave decision. You can't live your life for other people. You can't have a transplant to repay anyone – not your family or anyone else. In the end, you are the only one who can live your life – and choose when to stop doing that.'

'That's true,' he said. 'And although Mum may not think so now, in the end it will be better for her. This is no life for her either. I want her to be able to grieve for me and then get her life back. Do you think she'll be able to do that? Do you think a mother can ever get over losing a child?'

Penny didn't know how to answer this. He urgently needed her to say 'yes'. It was going to be important for his peace of mind. 'I'm not sure "get over it" is quite the right way to put it, Daniel,' she said. 'I think it's more that mothers find a place for the children they've lost, and that becomes a part of them and who they are – and then they make their lives again as slightly different people.' That seemed to satisfy him, because he nodded and fell silent. She was thankful that he didn't know about her own baby; he would never have asked her the question that was troubling him most.

Letting go

'The best New York book is there – up on the top shelf,' Daniel said. 'Help yourself.'

Penny's husband John was taking her to New York the next day for their twentieth wedding anniversary. Daniel had been there two years previously and over the past few days had enjoyed giving her the benefit of his wisdom on the best sights to visit.

'Thanks . . . got it,' Penny replied. She looked carefully at Daniel, who was lying on his bed, clearly exhausted and breathless. Over the five months since his decision not to have the transplant, he had deteriorated quite rapidly. But still, just yesterday he would have been able to get up and get the book for her.

'Daniel – you are quite a lot more breathless today. Have you had your nebuliser yet?'

'No, but don't worry – I'll be OK in a few minutes. You've just caught me after Mum has done my physio for me – I can't manage it myself now.'

'Does the physio help at all?'

'The truth? No, actually, it's a nightmare. It makes me feel completely knackered and breathless, and I feel bloody awful for about an hour afterwards.'

Penny came and sat on the edge of Daniel's bed. 'You know – if it's just making things worse for you, it is OK to stop doing it,' she said.

Daniel shook his head. 'I can't do that Penny,' he said. 'I have to keep going with it – for Mum and for Sara. If I stop, they'll know it's the end.'

'Would you like me to talk to them for you?' Penny asked.

'Thanks. Really thanks a lot. But no. I can deal with it,' Daniel said. 'But Penny, I did just want to say that it's been so good to have someone I can talk straight to about the hard stuff. Someone who won't fold up in tears like Mum and Sara.'

'Look Daniel . . . about New York . . .'

'You're going to have such a great time,' Daniel said before she could get any further. They talked for a while longer about the forthcoming trip, while Penny did a quick check of Daniel's drugs and supplies so that she could give a clear handover to the colleague who would be covering for her in her absence.

Downstairs, Susan was sitting at the kitchen table repotting a couple of house plants. It was a job she had been intending to do for ages, but now it served as a suitable distractor. She looked up in surprise when Sara came back in with Daniel's lunch tray.

'What's the matter?' she asked. 'Didn't he want it?'

'I didn't actually go in,' Sara replied. 'I got as far as the door, but he was having a sort of private conversation with Penny.'

Susan looked at her quizzically and then carried on patting compost down around an oversized spider plant. Sara sat down opposite her at the table.

'Mum, you know I said I'd come over and help Daniel with his physio tomorrow morning while you're at the dentist's?' she said. 'Well I was thinking that maybe he doesn't need it. It really makes him knackered you know.'

Susan didn't look up. 'Don't be daft,' she said. 'Of course he needs it. His lungs will fill up if he doesn't get it.'

'No Mum – you don't understand. I couldn't help overhearing what he was saying to Penny. Mum . . . he's wants to stop. He's only doing it for us.'

Susan finished arranging compost around the second plant, and went and washed her hands. She carefully replaced both pots on the window ledge and wiped the kitchen table. By the time she sat down again and took Sara's hand across the table, she was perfectly composed.

'You know, I think it's time for me to phone Matthew, and ask him to come and stay for a while', she said.

Penny moved Daniel's table back closer to his bed and topped up the water in his glass.

'Anything else you need?' she asked.

'No, fine thanks,' he replied. 'Mum's making me some lunch, I think, but I'm not very hungry.'

'OK, I'll be off then,' Penny said. She longed to kiss him goodbye, this boy she had known all his life. But she could never have done that at the best of times, and certainly not now, when he was a self-conscious fifteen-year-old. She knew that the one thing she had to do for Daniel now was to ensure that she didn't burden him with her own grief, when he was already having to cope with everyone else's. She had to maintain the calm, efficient, professional persona that he had always relied on.

She squeezed his hand. 'See you when I get back from New York.'

'Sure,' Daniel replied. They both knew it wasn't true, but they needed this very small lie to make the parting easier. Penny stepped out into the hall.

'Penny, one thing,' Daniel called. She knew it was an effort for him to raise his voice, and she came back quickly into the room. 'Will you pick me up 200 Silk Cut on your way back through Duty Free?'

As Penny got into her car, and dropped Daniel's guidebook onto the passenger seat, she realised that he had seen through her at the last. That parting shot had been his way of helping her. If she hadn't managed to fool him, she had to do better with John; he had been planning this trip for months and was determined to make it special for her. She glanced at herself in the rear mirror, reapplied her lipstick, and picked up her mobile phone to ring and tell him she was on her way home.

THE PATIENT'S JOURNEY: TRAVELLING THROUGH LIFE WITH A CHRONIC ILLNESS

A new BMJ series to deepen doctors' understanding

On 11 September 2004, the *BMJ* launched a new series, under the banner above. The editorial lead-in to the new series was as follows:

> For many years we have been keen to bring patients' voices into the *BMJ* by publishing personal views and commentaries by patients. Now we are starting a new intermittent series of longer articles describing patients' experiences of living with chronic disease. The first of these articles is published today, and we hope that readers will send us more along the same lines.

In response to this invitation, the following was submitted by Susan Johnson for publication in the *BMJ*. She is currently waiting to hear if it has been accepted.

Snakes and Ladders: my son's journey through health and illness

I have a photograph of my son Daniel on my desk at work. It was taken on the day he won the borough competition for Best Young Pianist of the Year. He is looking embarrassed and uncomfortable in his suit and clutching the certificate given to him by the Lady Mayoress. I used to have the picture on the sideboard at home, but Daniel always hated it and made me take it down . . . so I'm glad he doesn't know how many people see it every day now.

Today is a special day. It's Daniel's birthday. He would have been eighteen years old, but he died two and a half years ago. He had cystic fibrosis. I wish I could be out buying him an expensive present to mark his passing into manhood, but it was not to be. So instead I am spending his birthday weekend writing this article for the *BMJ*, because it is the only gift I can give to him and others like him. This is not going to be a sentimental article about my son – I mentioned the photograph only to establish that Daniel was a real person, with his own achievements and quirks. This article is about the NHS – and about what I have learned in the past eighteen years. I hope some of it will be of benefit to staff and patients, and help ease the journey of future Daniels.

I don't really remember much about the first six months after Daniel died – they were a blur. My husband Matthew had left me several years earlier and my daughter Sara was living with her boyfriend, so I was by myself. In the months before Daniel died, looking after him had become my whole life. I had had to give up work because he needed round-the-clock care. Then suddenly there was nothing – just this huge void and so many hours to fill each day. Eventually, I knew I had to find something to focus my mind, so I decided to finish the BA in management studies that I had started years earlier through the Open University. The work absorbed me and I finished the degree in just under a year. I got my current job as Outpatient Services Manager at St Michael's Hospital a couple of months later. In case it sounds like I am trying to pay back some kind of debt to the NHS, I'm not. I just wanted an interesting and challenging job; I had a fair bit of previous management experience in the commercial sector, and this was the first job that appealed to me.

I first heard about the 'Patient Journey' section of the *BMJ* a couple of weeks ago, when I met Dr Stebbing, our ex-GP, in the Outpatient Department. He retired last year on ill-health grounds because of bad angina and had come to see the cardiologist.[1] It was a very strange moment when we met – suddenly we were on opposite sides of the health-care fence: me on the inside and him on the outside. After his appointment, we had a coffee together and talked for a long time – and it was his advice and encouragement that made me decide to write this article.

---

1 I have Dr Stebbing's permission to share this information, and would like to dedicate this article to him, and to all the staff who looked after Daniel – as well as to Daniel himself.

It has taken me eighteen years to distil everything I have learned: first as a user of the NHS and now as a member of staff. Finally, I think I can sum it all up in a few sentences. I believe there are three crucial cornerstones that are the foundation for good health care: *communication, trust* and *shared decision-making*. The three are completely interdependent. You can't have trust without good communication, and you can't have shared decision-making without trust. At first, it sounds as if those foundations should be so easy to lay – but unfortunately there are three counter-forces working against them. They are *system complexity, resource pressure* and *uncertainty*. Each time one of those counter-forces comes into play, it undermines the cornerstones of care. Perhaps the best way for me to explain what I mean is through my journey with Daniel.

The moment you are told that your child has a life-threatening illness is etched on your memory forever. We were given that news catastrophically badly, by a junior doctor who was ill-prepared for the task. Part of the problem was that he had little experience of breaking such news to parents but, to a large degree, he was let down by a complex and overloaded system. As a newly appointed registrar, he should never have ended up by himself in a busy Outpatient Department without even having the necessary paperwork to hand – trying his best to impart information that was going to turn our lives upside down. That junior registrar was to become one of the foremost consultants at the Albion Children's Hospital and someone we would come to trust and rely on to ensure that Daniel had the best possible care. Although I didn't realise it then, that was the first time that I saw communication undermined by system complexity.

I think that for most of the next six months I was in a state of shock and grief. Daniel was very ill – he spent the majority of that time in the Albion – and I desperately needed some kind of security in a world that was unpredictable and frightening. I created that security for myself by coming to trust and rely on the doctors and nurses at the Albion. I relied on them to the exclusion of all else. In the end, when it came to Daniel's care, I didn't even trust myself, let alone my husband Matthew – who was doing his best to look my daughter Sara and maintain some semblance of normality in our lives. Communication between Matthew and myself became unbearably strained, and I was afraid that our marriage would break up.

There came a time when this could not go on any longer. Daniel had to come home, and Dr Stebbing, the local community team and St Michael's Hospital had to take responsibility for his medical care. I did everything I could to resist this change. I didn't know those people; I was uncertain about their ability to look after Daniel; and I wasn't prepared to trust them with my sick and fragile son. That was when I first met Penny, our community paediatric nurse. When you have a sick child, there are a few special people in your lives – the ones who really hold things together for you. Penny was one such person. She came to see me in the Albion and, in the end, I think she quite literally talked me out of there. I don't know how she had the patience, because it must have been like coaxing a rabbit out of its burrow. So much could have gone wrong during that transfer. Daniel had to come home on oxygen and getting everything organised was incredibly complicated. It meant that there had to be good communication between organisations, not just individuals. I think that if any part of the system had failed at that time, I'd have been back into my burrow like the frightened rabbit that I was. Fortunately, the system didn't fail – Penny had made sure of that – and so I gradually transferred my trust from the Albion to the local team. On that occasion, good communication triumphed over a complex system.

When I look back on those early days and think about communication, I know it's a two-way business. I'm sure I was a very difficult parent to deal with. Once I got past the grief, I was angry. It's a textbook pattern really, but I think I spent the next few years being angry with everyone and everything. If even the most trivial thing went wrong, I'd yell at someone or burst into tears. Maybe it was the only way I could be in control, but that's not really an excuse. I do remember one day shouting at some poor bed manager at the Albion, because Daniel was supposed to be going in for some investigations and they cancelled us at the last moment. Up to that time, the Albion could do no wrong in my eyes – and then suddenly they'd let us down. It was a huge blow to my trust in the hospital that I had believed could work miracles.

So this is where resource pressure – the next 'villain of the piece' –- comes in. I know now, from the other side of the fence, just what it's like juggling limited resources, and how that bed manager must have felt. For me, it's outpatient appointments rather than beds. I hate having to tell desperately anxious patients that there isn't an appointment available or, worse still on rare occasions, that their appointment has been cancelled. The biggest resource pressure in the NHS is staff – and staff pressure means time pressure. Time to explain, time to listen, time to fit in another appointment, time to go and see someone at home, time to coax a frightened mother out of a specialist hospital. In short, time to communicate well and to build trust.

Sometimes, these counter-forces can work together to create a really potent and dangerous mix. When Daniel was about nine, he was in the Albion with an infected portacath. On that occasion, we fell foul of both resource pressure and system complexity. It was a day when they were short of staff on the ward, and all sorts of things went wrong with the system. The safeguards failed and there was a drug error: Daniel was given too high a dose of his antibiotic. I completely lost control. In fact, I don't think anyone managed the situation very well – either the staff or myself. We all ended up shouting at each other and, for a long time, the trust that had been built up over so long was paper thin again.

In the end we all move on, and I gradually started to develop a more considered approach to Daniel's illness and a more reciprocal relationship with those looking after him. I think a landmark episode was when Daniel was eleven years old and needed to go on a trial of medicine that had only recently been used in children with cystic fibrosis. There was good evidence that it was effective in improving lung function in the short term, but no one was quite sure about the best longer-term dose or treatment regime – or even if there would be damaging side effects from chronic use. Up to that time, I'd really believed in the nebulous concept of a 'body of medical knowledge', like an enormous cook book with all the answers. Provided you went to the best experts, they would have those answers to hand. I know that sounds naïve. On another level, I'd seen enough documentaries about research and new developments to know that there were, and still are, many unanswered questions. Even so, part of the survival mechanism is to keep those two parts of your brain separate. So, for many years, my trust in Daniel's doctors was predicated on a personal pretence that they were omnipotent and could take the burden of decision-making away from me. I suspect that for many of my mother's generation, that belief still holds. So that was when I first realised – or more accurately first acknowledged – that the doctors don't have all the answers, that medicine is an inexact science – in fact, more of an art than a science – and is based on probabilities rather than facts.

I have to confess that at first I panicked. Uncertainty – the third 'villain' – was perhaps the most frightening of all. One can always believe that complex systems can be simplified by streamlining processes – and much of my current job is about doing just that. Even resource pressures can be tackled through greater investment and creative ways of working. But uncertainty will always be there and it demands of patients a more active role in directing the course of their illness. Doctors have been rightly criticised for being paternalistic, but if they are going to change this behaviour, then patients have to grow up and become mature partners. Patient autonomy has to be the right direction of travel, but it would be foolish to believe this is an easy journey – particularly when you are frightened and desperate for reassurance. In the end, I did become a mature partner, and the reason that was possible was that I had such a solid foundation of trust in Daniel's health-care team. The trust enabled me to deal with the uncertainty.

Trust and uncertainty are not just forces that are traded off in individual doctor–patient relationships. You only have to look at the fall-off in parents taking their children to have MMR vaccination or the anxiety about BSE and GM food to understand that. There has been a huge loss of trust in doctors and scientists. Apart from a few exceptional cases, that's not because they have been lying or deliberately distorting the facts. It's because their uncertainty has been exposed – the fact that they can talk in terms of very strong probabilities, but they can never say 'never'. They can't absolutely promise zero-risk from BSE, from GM foods or from MMR. The uncertainty has made people afraid about things that they didn't give a thought to previously – in the same way that I was afraid when I realised the doctors couldn't give me all the answers. Of course, sometimes doctors make things worse when they compound uncertainty by communicating it badly – by trying to hide the uncertainty behind arrogance instead of being honest about it. One thing I am grateful for is that none of the doctors looking after Daniel did that to me.

So finally, I thought I had reached the point in my journey where I could deal with Daniel's illness. I was ready to declare myself an 'expert parent'. Little did I know that the hardest step was yet to come. I had gone through a painful struggle to reach the stage where I could work in partnership with the clinical team and make informed choices about Daniel's care. Then quite suddenly one day, I was no longer the partner, and they were not my choices to make. They were Daniel's.

The day came long before I was ready for it, and the choice was a life-and-death one. Daniel's lung function had deteriorated badly and he needed a heart–lung transplant if he was to survive. I clung on to the hope of that transplant and never for one moment considered the possibility that Daniel might have a different view. He was only fifteen – how could he? But he did have a different view. He was braver than me and he chose to let go – and I had to respect his choice and recognise his autonomy, in the same way that the doctors had had to recognise mine.

What useful messages can health-care staff take away from this story? I think there are two things that I want to say.

First, my encounter with Dr Stebbing made me realise that the line between those giving and those receiving care is an artificial one. We all have a role to play in improving health – whether our own or someone else's. It's very easy to jump over the health-care fence – whether you are a member of staff who becomes ill or a patient who sets up a support group or joins a patient forum.

Second, I've thought a lot about these positive and negative forces, pulling in opposite directions. They seem to be like two concentric circles, the one locked inside the other. I think the Government has recognised some of the negative forces: the system failures, the underfunding and the way in which uncertainty has undermined public trust. I don't know if all their strategies for dealing with these problems are the right ones, but at least they've made a start.

The really important point is that I don't think it's the government policies that are the most powerful lever for turning those wheels in the right direction on a day-to-day basis. On every occasion where things went right for Daniel, it was the actions, commitment and motivation of the people at the front line that made the difference.

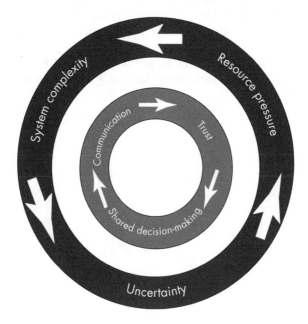

Figure 8.1 Positive and negative forces in health care.

Afterword

I have explained throughout this book that by today's standards Daniel was unlucky in the rate of progression of his illness and his early death. I 'let' him die at this early age to illustrate some important points about choice and autonomy.

Young people with cystic fibrosis can now expect to live into their thirties. Lung transplant increases survival by an average of four to five years, and survival rates are continuing to improve. Technically, it may be easier to transplant both the donor's heart and lungs into a patient with cystic fibrosis rather than the lungs alone. In this situation, because the heart of the cystic fibrosis patient is perfectly healthy, it can be given to another person, so that two people get a chance for life.

Without apology, I will end by giving details of UK Transplant's web site <http://www.uktransplant.org.uk> and telephone number (0845 60 60 400).

Bibliography

Abadie, A. and S. Gay, (2004) 'The Impact of Presumed Consent Legislation on Cadaveric Organ Donation: A Cross Country Study', *National Bureau of Economic Research*, Working Paper No. w10604.

Alaszewski, A. and T. Horlick-Jones (2003) 'How Can Doctors Communicate Information about Risk more Effectively?', *BMJ*, 327: 728–31.

Allen, I. (2001) 'Stress in Hospital Medicine: A Problem for Key Hospital Staff', *Hosp. Med.*, 62 (8): 501–3.

Audit Commission (2002) *Recruitment and Retention: A Public Service Workforce for the 21st Century*, London: Audit Commission for Local Authorities and the National Health Service in England and Wales.

Australian Law Reform Commission (1989) *Informed Decisions about Medical Procedures*, Canberra: ALRC.

Aynsley-Green, A., M. Barker, S. Burr, A. Macfarlane, J. Morgan, J. Sibert, T. Turner, R. Viner, T. Waterston and D. Hall (2000) 'Who is Speaking for Children and Adolescents and for Their Health at the Policy Level?', *BMJ*, 321: 229–32.

Aynsley-Green, A. (2002) *The Child First and Always: Is It?* Great Ormond Street Annual Lecture.

—— (2004) 'Is All Well with Children and Childhood and the Health-Related Services Provided for Them in Contemporary Society? 1. Historical Context and New Opportunities', *Current Paediatrics*, 14: 145–53.

Baggs, J. G., M. H. Schmitt, A. I. Mushlin, P. H. Mitchell, D. H. Eldredge, D. Oakes and A. D. Hutson (1999) 'Association between Nurse–Physician Collaboration and Patient Outcomes in Three Intensive Care Units', *Crit. Care Med.*, 27 (9): 1991–8.

Barach, P. and S. D. Small (2000) 'Reporting and Preventing Medical Mishaps: Lessons from Non-Medical Near Miss Reporting Systems', *BMJ*, 320: 759–63.

Becker, P. (Sept 2002) 'The Online Encyclopedia of Washington State History', History Link, <http://www.historylink.org/_output.CFM?file_ID=3928> (accessed 5 February 2005).

Blumstein, J. F. (1999) 'Legalizing Payment for Transplantable Cadaveric Organs', in H. Kuhse and P. Singer, eds, *Bioethics* Oxford: Blackwell Publishing, pp. 390–8.

Bolam v. *Friern Hospital Management Committee* [1957] 1 WLR 582.

Bolitho v. *City and Hackney Health Authority* [1997] 4 All ER 771.

Bolman, L. and T. Deal (1997) *Reframing Organizations: Artistry, Choice and Leadership*, San Francisco, CA: Wiley Press: Jossey-Bass Leadership Series.

Bridson, J., C. Hammond, A. Leach and M. R. Chester (2003) 'Making Consent Patient Centred', *BMJ*, 327: 1159–61.

Bristol Royal Infirmary Inquiry (2001) *Learning from Bristol: The Report of the Public Inquiry into Children's Heart Surgery at the Bristol Royal Infirmary*, Command Paper CM 5207, London: The Stationery Office.

British Medical Association (2001) *Withholding and Withdrawing Life-Prolonging Medical Treatment*, London: BMJ Books.

British Medical Association and Law Society (1995) 'Assessment of Mental Capacity: Guidance for Doctors and Lawyers' London: BMA.

British Medical Association and MORI (May 2004) 'Trust in Doctors: Omnibus Questions for 2004', Available online at <http://www.bma.org.uk/ap.nsf/Content/TrustInDocs2004> (accessed 5 February 2005).

Buchan, J. (2004) 'International Rescue? The Dynamics and Policy Implications of the International Recruitment of Nurses to the UK', *J. Health Serv. Res. Policy*, 9 (Suppl 1): 10–16.

Buchan, J. and N. Edwards (2000) 'Nursing Numbers in Britain: The Argument for Workforce Planning', *BMJ*, 320: 1067–70.

Bush, A. (2000) 'Guidelines for the Ethical Conduct of Medical Research Involving Children', *Arch. Dis. Child*, 83 (4): 370.

Calnan, M. W. and E. Sanford (2004) 'Public Trust in Health Care: The System or the Doctor?', *Qual. Saf. Health Care*, 13 (2): 92–7.

Capstick, B. (2004) 'The Future of Clinical Negligence Litigation?', *BMJ*, 328: 457–9.

Carvel, J. (2004) 'NHS Workforce Has More People than Birmingham', *Guardian*, 20 March.

Cass, H. D., I. Smith, C. Unthank, C. Starling and J. E. Collins (2003) 'Improving Compliance with Requirements on Junior Doctors' Hours', *BMJ*, 327: 270–3.

Cassell, E. J. (1976) *The Healer's Art: A New Approach to the Doctor–Patient Relationship*, New York: Lippincott.

Cystic Fibrosis Trust (2004) 'Are Patients with CF Getting a Fair Deal from the NHS?' *CF Today* (summer): 8.

Checkland, K., M. Marshall and S. Harrison (2004) 'Re-Thinking Accountability: Trust Versus Confidence in Medical Practice', *Qual. Saf. Health Care*, 13 (2): 130–5.

Chen, S. M. and A. McMurray (2001) '"Burnout" in Intensive Care Nurses', *J. Nurs. Res.*, 9 (5): 152–64.

Chester v. *Afshar* [2004] UKHL 41.

Coomarasamy, A. and K. S. Khan (2004) 'What is the Evidence that Postgraduate Teaching in Evidence Based Medicine Changes Anything? A Systematic Review', *BMJ*, 329: 1017.

Coulter, A. (1999) 'Paternalism or Partnership? Patients have Grown Up – and There's No Going Back', *BMJ*, 319: 719–20.

Craft, A. W. and D. M. Hall (2004) 'Munchausen Syndrome by Proxy and Sudden Infant Death', *BMJ*, 328: 1309–12.

Davis, C. (2003) 'Closed Minds', *Guardian*, 14 May.

Davies, C. (2000) 'Getting Health Professionals to Work Together', *BMJ*, 320: 1021–2.

Dekker, S. (2002) *The Field Guide to Human Error Investigations*, Aldershot: Ashgate.

Department for Education and Skills and Department of Health (2003) 'Every Child Matters' available online at <http://www.dfes.gov.uk/everychildmatters> (accessed 5 February 2005).

—— (2004) *National Service Framework for Children, Young People and Maternity Services*, London: DH Publications.

Department of Health (1989) *Working for Patients*, London: DH Publications.

—— (1997) *The New NHS, Modern, Dependable*, London: DH Publications.

—— (1998) *A First Class Service: Quality in the New NHS*, London: DH Publications.

—— (2000a) *A Health Service of All the Talents: Developing the NHS Workforce*, London: DH Publications.

—— (2000b) *An Organisation with a Memory*, London: DH Publications.

—— (2001a) *A Commitment to Quality, A Quest for Excellence*, London: DH Publications.

—— (2001b) *Shifting the Balance of Power*, London: DH Publications.

—— (2001c) *Good Practice in Consent Implementation Guide: Consent to Examination or Treatment*, London: DH Publications.

—— (2003a) *NHS Complaints Reform: Making Things Right*, London: DH Publications.

—— (2003b) *Keeping the NHS Local: A New Direction of Travel*, London: DH Publications.

—— (2003c) *NHS Modernisation Board Report*, 10 March.

—— (2004) *The Chief Executive's Report to the NHS 2004*, London: DH Publications.

—— (2005) 'Copying Letters to Patients', available on-line at <http://www.dh.gov.uk/PolicyAndGuidance/OrganisationPolicy/PatientAndPublicInvolvement/CopyingLettersToPatients/fs/en> (accessed 5 February 2005).

Dixon, J. (2001) 'Reforming Health Care, Saskatchewan Style', *Lancet*, 358 (9281): 526.

Donaldson, L. J. (1998) 'Clinical Governance: A Statutory Duty for Quality Improvement', *J. Epidemiol. Community Health*, 52 (2): 73–4.

—— (1999) 'Quality in Health Care: The US/UK Policy Perspectives', conference hosted by the Commonwealth Fund of New York and the Nuffield Trust, Ditchley Park, 21–23 May.

—— (2002) 'Intrathecal Chemotherapy', *Annual Report of the Chief Medical Officer*, London: DH Publications, pp. 46–53.

—— (2003) *Making Amends: A Consultation Paper Setting Out Proposals for Reforming the Approach to Clinical Negligence in the NHS*, London: DH Publications.

Edwards, P. (2004) 'Resource Allocation and the Right to Medical Treatment', *NHS Litigation Authority Review: Human Rights Special Issue*, vol. 30, pp. 6–7.

Edwards, N., M. Marshall, A. McLellan and K. Abbasi (2003) 'Doctors and Managers: A Problem without a Solution?', *BMJ*, 326: 609–10.

Enright M. (2004) '"Mature" Minors and The Medical Law: Safety First?', *Cork Online Law Review*, VII (3).

Equi, A., I. M. Balfour-Lynn, A. Bush and M. Rosenthal (2002) 'Long Term Azithromycin in Children with Cystic Fibrosis: A Randomised, Placebo-Controlled Crossover Trial', *Lancet*, 360 (9338): 978–84.

Erin, C. A. and J. Harris (2003) 'An Ethical Market in Human Organs', *J. Med. Ethics*, 29 (3): 137–8.

European Commission (2004) 'Commission Consultation on a Draft Proposal for a European Parliament and Council Regulation (EC) on Medicinal Products for Paediatric Use', available on-line at <http://pharmacos.eudra.org/F2/Paediatrics/index.htm> (accessed 5 February 2005).

Eysenbach, G. and A. R. Jadad (2001) 'Evidence-Based Patient Choice and Consumer Health Informatics in the Internet Age', *J. Med. Internet Res.*, 3 (2): E19.

Ferguson, T. and G. Frydman (2004) 'The First Generation of E-Patients', *BMJ*, 328: 1148–9.

Ferner, R. E. (2000) 'Medication Errors that Have Led to Manslaughter Charges', *BMJ*, 321: 1212–16.

Firth-Cozens, J. (2001) 'Cultures for Improving Patient Safety through Learning: The Role of Teamwork', *Qual. Saf. Health Care*, 10 (Suppl 2): ii26–ii31.

—— (2003) 'Doctors, Their Wellbeing, and Their Stress', *BMJ*, 326: 670–1.

—— (2004) 'Organisational Trust: The Keystone to Patient Safety', *Qual. Saf. Health Care*, 13 (1): 56–61.

Firth-Cozens, J., H. Cording and R. Ginsburg (2003) 'Can We Select Health Professionals who Provide Safer Care', *Qual. Saf. Health Care*, 12 (Suppl 1): i16–i20.

Fitzpatrick, M. (2004) 'The Cot Death Controversy', available online at <http://www.spiked-online.com/Articles/0000000CA3D8.htm> (accessed 5 February 2005).

Freedman, B. (1987) 'Equipoise and the Ethics of Clinical Research', *N. Engl. J. Med.*, 317 (3): 141–5.

Frenchay Healthcare NHS Trust v. *S* [1994] 1 WLR 601.

Gabbay, J. and A. le May (2004) 'Evidence Based Guidelines or Collectively Constructed "Mindlines?" Ethnographic Study of Knowledge Management in Primary Care', *BMJ*, 329: 1013.

Geneva International Labour Office (1999) *Terms of Employment and Working Conditions in Health Sector Reforms*, Geneva: ILO.

Gigerenzer, G. and A. Edwards (2003) 'Simple Tools for Understanding Risks: From Innumeracy to Insight', *BMJ*, 327: 741–4.

Gillick v. *West Norfolk and Wisbeach Health Authority* [1985] 3 All ER 402 (HL).

Glendinning, C., S. Kirk, A. Guiffrida and D. Lawton (2001) 'Technology-Dependent Children in the Community: Definitions, Numbers and Costs', *Child Care Health Dev.*, 27 (4): pp. 321–34.

Green, M. A. and S. Limerick (1999) 'For Debate: Time to Put "Cot Death" to Bed? Not Time to Put Cot Death to Bed?', *BMJ*, 319: 697–700.

Greenhalgh, T. (2000) *How to Read a Paper*, 6th edn, London: BMJ Books.

Hagger, L. E. (2004) 'The Human Rights Act 1998 and Medical Treatment: Time for Re-Examination', *Arch. Dis. Child*, 89 (5): 460–3.

Ham, C. (1999) 'Tragic Choices in Health Care: Lessons from the Child B Case', *BMJ*, 319: 1258–61.

Hammond, P. (2003) 'Risky Business', Primary Care, available on-line at <http://www.nhs.uk/nhsmagazine/primarycare/archives/feb2003/signin g.asp> (accessed 5 February 2005).

Harris, J. and C. Erin (2002) 'An Ethically Defensible Market in Organs', *BMJ*, 325: 114–15.

Hartmann, L. C., D. J. Schaid, J. E. Woods, T. P. Crotty, J. L. Myers, P. G. Arnold, P. M. Petty, T. A. Sellers, J. L. Johnson, S. K. McDonnell, M. H. Frost and R. B. Jenkins (1999) 'Efficacy of Bilateral Prophylactic Mastectomy in Women with a Family History of Breast Cancer', *N. Engl. J. Med.*, 340 (2): 77–84.

Health Canada (2001) *Talking Tools II: Putting Communication Skills to Work* (Course Book), on-line publication, p. 11.

Healthcare Commission (2004) 'State of Healthcare Report', available on-line at <http://www.healthcarecommission.org.uk> (accessed 5 February 2005).

Helman, C. (2003) *Culture, Health and Illness*, 4th edn, London: Hodder Arnold.

Holbrook, J. (2003a) 'The Trouble with Making Amends', *Spiked Online*, available on-line at <http://www.spiked-online.com/articles/00000006DEDE. htm> (accessed 5 February 2005).

—— (2003b) 'The Criminalisation of Fatal Medical Mistakes', *BMJ*, 327: 1118–19.

Horbar, J. D., J. H. Carpenter, J. Buzas, R. F. Soll, G. Suresh, M. B. Bracken, L. C. Leviton, P. E. Plsek and J. C. Sinclair (2004) 'Collaborative Quality Improvement to Promote Evidence Based Surfactant for Preterm Infants: A Cluster Randomised Trial', *BMJ*, 329: 1004.

Horrocks, S., E. Anderson and C. Salisbury (2002), 'Systematic Review of Whether Nurse Practitioners Working in Primary Care Can Provide Equivalent Care to Doctors', *BMJ*, 324: 819–23.

Horton, R. (2004) 'Why is Ian Kennedy's Healthcare Commission Damaging NHS Care?', *Lancet*, 364: 401–2.

Humber, M. (2004) 'National Programme for Information Technology', *BMJ*, 328: 1145–46.

Iles, V. and K. Sutherland (2001) *Organisational Change: A Review for Health Care Managers, Professionals and Researchers*, London: NCCSDO.

Irvine, D. H. (2003) *The Doctors' Tale: Professionalism and Public Trust*, Oxford: Radcliffe Medical Press.

—— (2004) 'Time for Hard Decisions on Patient-Centred Professionalism', *Med. J. Aust.*, 181 (5): 271–4.

Jadad, A. R., C. A. Rizo and M. W. Enkin (2003) 'I Am a Good Patient, Believe It or Not', *BMJ*, 326: 1293–5.

Jenkins, I. (2004) 'The James Lind Legacy: The Past: James Lind', in M. Rawlins and P. Littlejohns, eds, *Delivering Quality in the NHS 2004*, Oxford: Radcliffe Medical Press, pp. 3–4.

Jones, A., P. Penfold, M. Bailey, C. Charig, D. Choolun and A. M. Rollin (2000) 'Pre-Admission Clerking of Urology Patients by Nurses', *Prof. Nurse*, 15 (4): 261–6.

Jones, J. W. (2000) 'The Healthcare Professional and the Bolam Test', *Br. Dent. J.*, 188 (5): 237–40.

Kirk, S. and C. Glendinning (2004) 'Developing Services to Support Parents Caring for a Technology-Dependent Child at Home', *Child Care Health Dev.*, 30 (3): 209–18.

Kitson, A., C. McManus and M. Pringle (1996) 'A Research Base for Professional Staffing in Health Services,' in M. Peckham, ed., *The Scientific Basis of Health Services*, London: BMJ Books, pp. 106–7.

Klein, R. (1991) 'On the Oregon Trail: Rationing Health Care', *BMJ*, 302 (6767): 1–2.

Kluge E.-H. W. (1999) 'Organ Donation and Retrieval: Whose Body is it Anyway?', in H. Kuhse and P. Singer, eds, *Bioethics*, Oxford: Blackwell Publishing, pp. 387–9.

Kurtz, S. M. and J. D. Silverman (1996) 'The Calgary-Cambridge Referenced Observation Guides: An Aid to Defining the Curriculum and Organizing the Teaching in Communication Training Programmes', *Med. Educ.*, 30 (2): 83–9.

Lamb, R. (2004) 'Open Disclosure: The Only Approach to Medical Error', *Qual. Saf. Health Care*, 13 (1): 3–5.

Laming (2003) The Victoria Climbié Inquiry, available on-line at <http://www.victoria-climbie-inquiry.org.uk> (accessed 5 February 2005).

Lock, D. (2002) 'Kidderminster: What Happens if It All Goes Wrong?', Presentation at *RCPCH Policy Conference*, 30 January, London: RCPCH.

Lockwood, D., M. Armstrong and A. Grant (2004) 'Integrating Evidence Based Medicine into Routine Clinical Practice: Seven Years' Experience at the Hospital for Tropical Diseases, London', *BMJ*, 329: 1020–3.

Lutchman, R. (2003) 'Pull Up Your Socks or Have Them Pulled Up for You', in *Rapid Responses, Electronic BMJ*, available on-line at <http://bmj.bmjjournals.com/cgi/eletters/327/7424/1118#41799> (accessed 5 February 2005).

Maguire, P. and C. Pitceathly (2002) 'Key Communication Skills and How to Acquire Them', *BMJ*, 325: 697–700.

Managing DNAs (2003) *NHS Management Briefing*, July, available on-line at <http://www.nelh.nhs.uk/management/mantop/0110dna.doc> (accessed 5 February 2005).

Marks, N. (2003) 'An Expert Witness Falls from Grace', *BMJ*, 327: 110.

Martineau, T., K. Decker and P. Bundred (2002) 'Briefing Note on International Migration of Health Professionals: Levelling the Playing Field for Developing Country Health Systems', Liverpool: Liverpool School of Tropical Medicine.

Marvel, M. K., R. M. Epstein, K. Flowers and H. B. Beckman (1999) 'Soliciting the Patient's Agenda: Have We Improved?', *JAMA*, 281 (3): 283–7.

Maynard, A., K. Bloor and N. Freemantle (2004) 'Challenges for the National Institute for Clinical Excellence', *BMJ*, 329: 227–9.

Maynard v. *West Midlands Health Authority* [1985] 1 All ER 635.

Medical Research Council (2004) *MRC Ethics Guide: Medical Research Involving Children*, London: Medical Research Council.

Michaud, P. A., J. C. Suris and R. Viner (2004) 'The Adolescent with a Chronic Condition. Part II: Healthcare Provision', *Arch. Dis. Child*, 89 (10): 943–9.

Milburn, A. (2002) Speech to the HR in the NHS Conference', 2 July.

—— (2003) Statement to the House of Commons by Secretary of State for Health Alan Milburn, on the publication of the Victoria Climbié Inquiry, 28 January.

Mill J. S. (1859) 'On Liberty', in H. Kuhse and P. Singer, eds, *Bioethics*, Oxford: Blackwell Publishing, pp. 515–16.

Modernisation Agency (2002) *Improvement Leaders' Guide to Involving Patients and Carers*, London: DH Publications.

Mullally, S. (2003), Keynote Address, Chief Nursing Officer Conference, November, Brighton.

NHS Confederation (2001a) *Why Won't the NHS Do as It Is Told – And What Might We Do About It?* London.

NHS Confederation (2001b) *Clinical Networks: A Discussion Paper*, London.

—— (2004) *NHS Management: Exploding the Myths*, London.

NHS Executive (2000) *The NHS Plan: A Plan for Investment. A Plan for Reform*. London: DH Publications.

North West Lancashire Health Authority v. *A, D and G* [2000] 1 WLR 977.

Nyatanga, L. (1998) 'Professional Ethnocentrism and Shared Learning', *Nurse Educ. Today*, 18 (3): pp. 175–7.

Nyatanga, L. and D. Forman (2002) 'Interprofessional Education (IPE): The Need for a Paradigm Shift', Capita Conference '*Developing the Infrastructure to Implement Lifelong Learning*', London, 19 June.

Otton, Lord Justice Philip (2001) 'Medical Negligence: Is There Something Wrong?', *Med. Leg. J.*, 69 (Pt 2): 72–84.

Paling, J. (2003) 'Strategies to Help Patients Understand Risks', *BMJ*, 327: 745–8.

Papadopoulos, M. C., M. Hadjitheodossiou, C. Chrysostomou, C. Hardwidge and B. A. Bell (2001) 'Is the National Health Service at the Edge of Chaos?', *J. R. Soc. Med.*, 94 (12): 613–16.

Parish, C. (2004) 'Take a Little More Time', *Nursing Standard*, 18 (45): 14–16.

Pearce v. United Bristol Healthcare NHS Trust [1999] PIQR 53.

Pearson, R., P. Reilly and D. Robinson (2004) 'Recruiting and Developing an Effective Workforce in the British NHS', *J. Health Serv. Res. Policy*, 9 (Suppl 1): 17–23.

Plsek, P. E. and T. Greenhalgh (2001) 'Complexity Science: The Challenge of Complexity in Health Care', *BMJ*, 323 (7313): 625–8.

Psirides, A. (2003) 'Re: Pull Up Your Socks or Have Them Pulled Up For You', *Rapid Responses, Electronic BMJ* http://bmj.bmjjournals.com/cgi/letters/327/7424/1118#41902 (accessed 17 July 2005).

Public fails to cancel appointments (1999) *BBC Online*, available on-line at <http://news.bbc.co.uk/1/hi/health/423052.stm> (accessed 5 February 2005).

Ramirez, A., J. Addington-Hall and M. Richards (1998) 'ABC of Palliative Care. The Carers', *BMJ*, 316 (7126): 208–11.

Rawlins, M. D. (1999) Speech by Professor Sir Michael Rawlins to St Paul International Health Care Annual Lecture, 7 September, available on-line at http://www.nice.org.uk/page.aspx?0=27856 (accessed 17 July 2005).

Rawlins, M. D. and A. J. Culyer (2004) 'National Institute for Clinical Excellence and its Value Judgments', *BMJ*, 329: 224–7.

Re C [1994] 1 FLR 31.

Re E [1993] 1 FLR 386.

Re L [1998] 2 FLR 810.

Re M [1999] 2 FLR 1097.

Re T [1992] 9 BMLR 46.

Reason, J. T. (2000) 'Human Error: Models and Management', *BMJ*, 320 (7237): 768–70.

Reason, J. T., J. Carthey and M. R. de Leval (2001) 'Diagnosing "Vulnerable System Syndrome": An Essential Prerequisite to Effective Risk Management', *Qual. Health Care*, 10 (Suppl 2): ii21–ii25.

Robertson v. Nottingham Health Authority [1997] 8 Med LR 1.

Rogers v. Whittaker [1992] 175 CLR 479.

Royal College of Paediatrics and Child Health (1997) *Withholding or Withdrawing Life Saving Treatment in Children. A Framework for Practice*, London: RCPCH.

Sackett, D. L., W. M. Rosenberg, J. A. Gray, R. B. Haynes and W. S. Richardson, (1996) 'Evidence Based Medicine: What It Is and What It Isn't', *BMJ* 312 (7023): 71–2.

Samanta, A. and J. Samanta (2003) 'Legal Standard of Care: A Shift from the Traditional Bolam Test', *Clin. Med.*, 3 (5): 443–6.

Scherer, P. (2004) 'Migration and the Global Healthcare Workforce: Balancing Competing Demands', San Diego, Calif., Academy Health's Annual Research

Meeting, available online at <http://www.academyhealth.org/2004/ppt/scherer.ppt> (accessed 5 February 2005).

Scottish Office (1998) *Managed Clinical Networks*, Scotland: Health Management Library, available on-line at http://www.scotland.gov.uk/deleted/library/documents5/acute-00.htm

Shaw, M. (2001) 'Competence and Consent to Treatment in Children and Adolescents', *Advances in Psychiatric Treatment*, 7: 150–9.

Shekelle, P. (2003) 'New Contract for General Practitioners', *BMJ*, 326: 457–8.

Sidaway v. Board of Governors of the Bethlem Royal Hospital and The Maudsley Hospital [1985] 1 All ER 643.

Silverman, W. A. (2003) 'Personal Reflections on Lessons Learned from Randomised Trials involving Newborn Infants, 1951–1967', available on-line at <http://www.jameslindlibrary.org> (accessed 5 February 2005).

Sinclair, R. and A. Franklin (2000) *A Quality Protects Research Briefing: Young People's Participation*. Department of Health: Research in Practice and Making Research Count.

Smith, J. (2000) 'A Register of Blunders or Botchers?', *BMJ*, 320 (7251): 1738.

—— (2004) *Shipman Inquiry. Safeguarding Patients: Lessons from the Past – Proposals for the Future*, 5th report, available at <http://www.the-shipman-inquiry.org.uk/fifthreport.asp> (accessed 5 February 2005).

Smith, J., K. Walshe and D. J. Hunter (2001) 'The "Redisorganisation" of the NHS', *BMJ*, 323: 1262–3.

Smith, L. and H. Daughtrey (2000) 'Weaving the Seamless Web of Care: An Analysis of Parents' Perceptions of Their Needs Following Discharge of Their Child From Hospital', *J. Adv. Nurs.*, 31 (4): 812–20.

Smith, R. (1998) 'All Changed, Changed Utterly. British Medicine will be Transformed by the Bristol Case', *BMJ*, 316: 1917–18.

—— (2000) 'The Failings of NICE', *BMJ*, 321: 1363–4.

—— (2003) 'Communicating Risk: The Main Work of Doctors', *BMJ*, 327: 0–f.

—— (2005) 'The GMC: Expediency Before Principle', *BMJ*, 330: 1–2.

Spencer, A. and S. Cropper (2004) 'Establishing Managed Clinical Networks in Paediatric Services: Experience of Partners in Paediatrics', *Current Paediatrics*, 14: 347–53.

Stanton, J. and A. Simpson (2001) 'Murder Misdiagnosed as SIDS: A Perpetrator's Perspective', *Arch. Dis. Child*, 85 (6): 454–9.

'Stress and General Practice' (2002) *Information Sheet 22*, Royal College of General Practitioners, available on-line at <http://www.rcgp.org.uk> (accessed 5 February 2005).

Sutcliffe, A. G. (2003) 'Testing New Pharmaceutical Products in Children', *BMJ*, 326: 64–5.

Tan, J. O. and J. R. McMillan (2004) 'The Discrepancy between the Legal Definition of Capacity and the British Medical Association's Guidelines', *J. Med. Ethics*, 30 (5): 427–9.

Tännsjö, T. (1999) 'The Morality of Clinical Research: A Case Study', in H. Kuhse and P. Singer, eds, *Bioethics*, Oxford: Blackwell Publishing, pp. 449–56.

Teuten, B. and D. Taylor (2001) '"Don't Worry my Good Man – You Won't Understand our Medical Talk": Consent to Treatment Today', *Br. J. Ophthalmol.*, 85 (8): 894–6.

Thom, D. H. (2001) 'Physician Behaviors that Predict Patient Trust', *J. Fam. Pract.*, 50 (4): 323–8.

Thom, D. H., R. L. Kravitz, R. A. Bell, E. Krupat and R. Azari (2002) 'Patient Trust in the Physician: Relationship to Patient Requests', *Fam. Pract.*, 19 (5): 476–83.

Towle, A. and W. Godolphin (1999) 'Framework for Teaching and Learning Informed Shared Decision Making', *BMJ*, 319: 766–71.

'Trust' (Dec 2002) Bandolier, available on-line at <http://www.jr2.ox.ac.uk/bandolier/booth/mgmt/trust.html> (accessed 5 February 2005).

Twistington Higgins, T. (1952) *Great Ormond Street 1852–1952*, London: Odhams Press.

Tyrrell, J. (2001) 'Growing up with Cystic Fibrosis: The Adolescent Years,' in M. Bluebond-Langner, B. Lask and D. B. Angst (eds) *Psychosocial Aspects of Cystic Fibrosis*, London: Arnold, pp. 139–49.

UK Transplant (2004a) 'Transplants Save Lives', available on-line at <http://www.uktransplant.org.uk/ukt/newsroom/fact_sheets/transplants_save_lives.jsp> (accessed 5 February 2005).

—— (2004b) 'National Potential Donor Audit', available on-line at <http://www.uktransplant.org.uk/ukt/statistics/potential_donor_audit/pdf/poster_apr03-may04.pdf> (accessed 5 February 2005).

Van der Dennen, J. (1985) 'Of Badges, Bonds and Boundaries: Ingroup/Outgroup Differentiation and Ethnocentrism', 5th Annual Meeting of the European Sociobiological Society, St John's College, Oxford, available on-line at <http://rint.rechten.rug.nl/rth/dennen/ethnocen.htm> (accessed 5 February 2005).

Walton, M. (2004) 'Creating a "No Blame" Culture: Have We Got the Balance Right?', *Qual. Saf. Health Care*, 13 (3): 163–4.

Wang, K. W. and A. Barnard (2004) 'Technology-Dependent Children and their Families: A Review', *J. Adv. Nurs.*, 45 (1): 36–46.

Weijer, C., S. H. Shapiro and G. K. Cranley (2000) 'For and Against: Clinical Equipoise and Not the Uncertainty Principle is the Moral Underpinning of the Randomised Controlled Trial', *BMJ*, 321: 756–8.

Whitehouse v. *Jordan* [1981] 1 All ER 267.

Wilsher v. *Essex Area Health Authority* [1988] AC 1074 (HL).

Woods, K. (2001) 'The Prevention of Intrathecal Medication Errors: A Report to the Chief Medical Officer', London: DH Publications.

Index

Note: page numbers in italics refer to figures or tables; names in italics refer to fictitious characters.

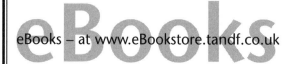